NURSING HISTORY
New Perspectives, New Possibilities

NURSING HISTORY
New Perspectives, New Possibilities

ELLEN CONDLIFFE LAGEMANN, Editor
Teachers College, Columbia University

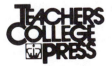

Teachers College, Columbia University
New York and London   1983

Published by Teachers College Press, 1234 Amsterdam Avenue,
New York, N.Y. 10027

Library of Congress Cataloging in Publication Data
Main entry under title:

Nursing history.

    Papers from a conference held May 1981, sponsored by the Rockefeller Archive
Center.
    Includes bibliographical references and index.
    1. Nursing—History—Congresses.   2. Nursing—United States—History—Con-
gresses.   I. Lagemann, Ellen Condliffe, 1945–   .   II. Rockefeller Archive Center.
[DNLM: 1. History of nursing—Congresses. WY 11.1 N974 1981]
RT31.N87   1983   610.73'09   82–10320

ISBN 0–8077–2730–X

Manufactured in the United States of America
88 87 86 85 84 83   1 2 3 4 5 6

Contents

Acknowledgments

This book would not have been possible without the generous support of the Rockefeller Archive Center, and I should especially like to thank Joseph W. Ernst, director of the Archive Center, and J. William Hess, associate director, for their generosity, interest, and advice.

Many people contributed to the conference, hosted by the Rockefeller Archive Center, for which the essays in this book were originally prepared. Louise Fitzpatrick, dean of the College of Nursing at Villanova University, Patricia Fry, associate professor and chairperson, Department of Research and Theory Development in Nursing Science, School of Nursing, New York University, and Marjorie J. Ramphal, acting director, Graduate Program, Columbia University School of Nursing, made invaluable suggestions at the first planning session. Lawrence A. Cremin, president of Teachers College and a member of the Governing Council of the Archive Center, helped to bring us all together and encouraged the publication of this book. Barbara J. Stevens, director of the Division of Health Services, Sciences, and Education and chairman of the Department of Nursing Education at Teachers College, shared in all aspects of the work that preceded the meeting—without her, the conference would not have been a success. In addition to those whose papers are presented here, the following people made presentations to the conference: Virginia Lieson Brereton (Teachers College), Ginny Durrin (Durrin Films), Wanda C. Heistad (New York University), Sydney Krampitz (University of Chicago), Judy Barret Litoff (Bryant College), Christopher Maggs (Bath, Avon, U.K.), Dorothy Sheahan (University of Pennsylvania), and Rosemary White (University of Manchester, U.K.). The late Teresa E. Christy (University of Iowa), Janet Wilson James (Boston College), Philip A. Kalish (University of Michigan), Charles E. Rosenberg (University of Pennsylvania), and Morris J. Vogel

(Temple University) served as commentators. Along with the other invited participants, all of these people contributed significantly to two days of lively discussion.

Finally, special thanks are owed to Janet Wilson James and Charles Rosenberg, who were extraordinarily generous in offering advice and comments at various stages in the planning of the conference and the preparation of this book.

—E.C.L.

NURSING HISTORY
New Perspectives, New Possibilities

1

INTRODUCTION
Nursing History: New Perspectives, New Possibilities

Ellen Condliffe Lagemann

In May 1981 the Rockefeller Archives Center in Pocantico Hills, New York, sponsored a two-day conference on the history of nursing. As the repository for the papers of the various Rockefeller philanthropies, the Archive Center hoped to encourage research in one of the areas in which it has extensive holdings. A number of American and British historians, archivists, and educators interested in nursing were therefore invited to the Archive Center to present and talk about recent work. Soon thereafter it was also decided to publish a number of the conference papers. In themselves, the essays seemed to warrant wider dissemination, and the Archive Center meeting had suggested that a collection of this kind might be valuable in promoting more general discussion of "needs and opportunities" within the field.

Often useful, such discussion is particularly warranted now because the history of nursing is very much in ferment. It is an area of research that is undergoing change in several significant ways. Once studied primarily by leaders in the profession, nursing history is now studied by scholars of diverse training and orientation. Principally concerned in the past with recording advances and achievements, nursing history now deals also with the sources, the problems, and the processes of occupational growth and change. The people, the organizations, the settings, and the events that have dominated the historiography of nursing throughout the century have not been set aside. But data once mined primarily to answer questions of professional lineage and descent are now additionally used to investigate larger and more general issues of social, economic, political, and cultural change.

Broadening in perspective and becoming increasingly varied in approach, nursing history is at an interesting and important point in its development. More than ever before, an area of research that touches upon matters of concern to many different people appears to be breaking out of the confines that have tended to obscure its wide relevance. Why that is happening, and happening now, is difficult to know, although two phenomena have undoubtedly contributed to the emergence of new styles and more complex questions.

Nursing is a field in which women are a majority, and growing interest in women's history has obviously fostered wider interest in nursing history. Further, as the problematics of women's history—its central questions and the criteria for measuring significance and relevance that determine what those questions shall be—has changed, questions derived from women's history and informed by women's history have begun to generate new kinds of queries to put to nursing's past.

Until relatively recently, women's history and nursing history were much the same in approach. In the 1960s and early 1970s, retrieving "notable" women from obscurity and calling attention to the events and movements that had helped to move women into public arenas and to gain for them progressively more access to traditionally male rights, powers, and activities defined the focus of both fields. Since that time, however, women's history has become more and more concerned with questions built around an awareness that public achievements, public politics, and public lives are not necessarily the only or the most fruitful aspects of history to examine in reconstructing the experience of women as individuals or as a social group. In other words, the initial realization that women have been invisible in history, as traditionally conceived, has led to the further realization that women can only become fully visible if traditional concepts, modes of analysis, and sources of data are, in many cases, modified, and in some, set aside. Hence, as early studies and continuing efforts to understand the meaning of feminism, generally and within history, have promoted more articulate and varied views of what gender difference implies, work in women's history has tended to leave behind the emphasis on "notableness" and "progress" that marked its initial resurgence almost twenty years ago. The greater sophistication with which scholars today investigate women's history and incorporate feminist perspectives into all kinds of research is, not surprisingly, now also more evident in specialized studies of women and work.[1]

If women's history has provided one spur to new views of nursing history, what may be called "the new historiography of professions" has provided a second. Of late, the development of many different professions has been scrutinized by scholars. Moreover, the limitations of narrowly defined, "insider"-oriented approaches to the history of professions and professional activities have been noted.

In some cases, new work has been concerned with the validity and usefulness of "standard" historical accounts. As is well known, that has been true in education. There, the realization that an unvarying emphasis on schools and schooling was anachronistic and had eclipsed the possibility of inquiring into the larger and more important process of cultural transmission across the generations has had clear effect. It has also been truly liberating to recognize that interpretations of educational history that invariably stressed universal benefit and social progress had obscured the complex, sometimes contradictory, and not always disinterested purposes and outcomes of education. Far more than was true before the 1960s, educational history is conceived as the study of a complicated and varied process that has mirrored and can tell much about changing capacities, technologies, and values.[2]

In medicine the shortcomings of internally oriented, uncritical accounts have also been noted and more contextual, less presentist work is far more common there also than it was in the past. Beyond that, in medicine, as in education, disenchantment with current practices and current politics has provoked studies of "the underside" of what was once portrayed as medical "progress." Works of this kind in both medicine and education have been criticized for sometimes veering in the direction of polemic and, on occasion, coming close to substituting overly simple "bleak" pictures for overly simple "rosy" ones. Such criticisms notwithstanding, the skepticism so injected into these historiographies has provided a much needed corrective to earlier pieties, while also raising innovative questions.[3]

Not only in medicine and in education, but in other areas as well, new work has grown out of the realization that there are significant relationships to be explored between the growth of professions, on the one hand, and contemporary transformations in culture, politics, and the economy, on the other; and that realization, in turn, has grown out of or at least been supported by changes in labor history, which no longer deals primarily with the history of unions and unionism, but more generally with the organization of work settings, work relationships, and work routines as integral aspects of cultural and social structures. Thus, causative links have been investigated between the professionalization of the social sciences at the turn of the century, growing and changing per-

ceptions of social problems, diminishing credence in traditionally au--
thoritative means for understanding and acting upon those problems,
and the development of more formally organized and rationalized settings for intellectual work; correspondences have been studied between
the emergence of engineering as a profession and the emergence of the
United States as a highly industrialized capitalist society, designed with
and by the knowledge and techniques of "engineers"; and connections
have been studied between the personal and collective needs of late-
nineteenth-century "child savers" and early definitions of and structures
for social work.[4]

New studies of the professions have often been informed by insights
drawn from sociology. Whether one defines a profession as a collegial
community based on commonly held esoteric knowledge, as an occupational group that shares an altruistic guardianship over the ethics and
performance standards of a vital social service, as a monopoly-seeking
and monopoly-maintaining guild, or merely as "something" everyone
wants to belong to, there is now historical work that at least implicitly
applies, and can be used explicitly to test, the validity of one's theoretical
view. Equally important, new studies have clarified, and may be expected
further to illuminate, the overall importance and the many functions of
professions as organizing structures for "modern" societies.[5]

One could go on, for "the new historiography of professions" is
abundant in quantity, varied in origin, richly diverse in point of view,
and highly integrated with and meaningful for investigations of both
historical questions and matters of present concern in public policy.
Even to describe the literature to which I am referring as "a new historiography" may suggest a unity that does not exist. In fact, one of the
fascinating things about recent studies of professionalization, the professions, and professional services, practices, politics, and knowledge do-
mains is the way these studies have cut across scholarly disciplines, and
perhaps for that reason seem to have the potential to lead toward new
historical syntheses. However that may be, it is useful here to speak of "a
new historiography of professions" in order to indicate a second source
of the more contextual, open-ended, critical, and sociologically informed
questions now evident in the history of nursing.

Of course, first to point out that nursing history is changing, and
then to suggest several reasons for those changes is simply to highlight
what may be observed by reading the essays in this book. What may not
be so readily apparent, however, is what new perspectives auger in terms
of possibilities for future work. Which of many research questions, de-
signs, and strategies will turn out to be most productive cannot yet, if

ever, be surely predicted. But what is already clear is that there are widely significant problems that future work can inform, *if*, through individual and collective reflection and conversation, the implications of past, present, and future historiographical choices are continuously, self-consciously, and searchingly reviewed.

One such problem has to do with the organization of work, in the past and today. Relative to some kinds of work and most kinds of "women's work," domestic and nondomestic, paid and unpaid, nursing is highly organized, closely controlled through education and licensing, grounded in knowledge and in an altruistic ethics—in short, very professionalized. Relative to the paradigmatic, traditionally male professions of medicine and law, by contrast, nursing is only incompletely professionalized or partially professionalized. With education and social work, among others, it is but a "semi-profession."[6]

The very terms used to describe "major professions," such as medicine, on the one hand, and "minor professions," such as nursing, on the other, are value-laden and in many ways misleading. At best, they point toward only one aspect of what needs to be known about nursing: its relationship to differently organized and differently valued lines of work. What is more, they reflect only one perspective on nursing's past: that of the women (and men) who have aspired to bring to nursing the kind of high standards, dignity, and autonomy they have believed it deserved. But what else needs to be known about nursing—about the services nurses have provided before and after their skills were professionally recognized; the social structures they have created, transformed, and operated within; the formal, intuitive, and experiential knowledge they have and have not developed and used; the roles they have assumed and been assigned as well as been denied; and the meanings they have and have not found in and through their work? And what other perspectives need to be added to and mixed with those of the elite?[7]

It is difficult to answer these questions, as it also is difficult to put them well; for, as our vocabulary testifies, our vision has been and is still unfortunately myopic and one-dimensional. Clearly, however, if nursing is significant on its own terms, whatever those terms, in fact, may be, it also deserves to be *studied* on its own terms. Yet what those terms are remains elusive, and shall have to be discovered through the accumulation of more knowledge, the use of a greater variety of vantage points, and the cultivation of heightened historiographical self-consciousness. To deal only or even primarily with those matters that illuminate nursing's likenesses or lack of likenesses to "major professions" may be woefully inadequate, although such investigations, enhanced with attentiveness to their inevitable shortcomings, eventually may lead to the development of a vocabulary and the vision necessary to describe the work of nurses—and many other people—in ways that are accurate to all of the varied and complex characteristics of such work. Certainly this problem of vocabulary and vision is one that future studies in nursing history can approach with benefit to any number of historical and policy questions.

Different from the above, but related to it, is a problem of audience and style. The opportunity in nursing history to develop a more fully and accurately descriptive vocabulary of work exemplifies the possibility now present to contribute to more fields of knowledge than nursing history traditionally has done. That possibility certainly promises much, and yet, to be realized it may require more theoretical, contextual, and critical kinds of analyses than have heretofore predominated in the field. Will?—must?—such analyses jeopardize the special and established value of nursing history to nurses themselves?

Beginning perhaps with M. Adelaide Nutting and Lavinia Dock's 1907 study, nursing history has provided a much needed source of information and inspiration to nursing students and nursing practitioners: models to emulate, earlier struggles to consider, ideals to share. And, at least in part, it has been able to serve this function because vivid and concrete details, sure lines of development, and contrasts with the present have given a drama, clarity, and immediacy to the history. Those qualities may be a sine qua non in making historical literatures interesting and valuable to mostly nonhistorian audiences. The problem, then, is to determine whether or not and how the kinds of questions, data, and styles that have traditionally created a "usable past" for nurses can be merged with the kinds of questions, data, and styles that could make nursing history in the future an equally "usable past" for non-nurses.[8]

Obviously the problem of addressing different audiences with different interests and needs is not a unique problem in nursing history. In educational history, for example, the same problem exists. Revisionist work in educational history since the 1960s has undoubtedly resulted in a more profound and rigorous scholarship according to the canons of craftsmanship of the historical profession. But whether or not that scholarship has been more useful, or even as useful, to practitioners in education is a serious question. Educational historians might say that it should have been more useful: according to the standards of their profession, it is a "better" history, a less anachronistic and less eulogistic history. Granted that, however, has this "better" educational history been sufficiently directed toward the questions of practice and the diurnal realities with which educators in the field are constantly confronted? Or have challenges to the professional biases of "educationists" simply resulted in those biases having been replaced with the biases of a different profession? The question has not been studied in a systematic way, but it does seem likely that the problems involved in mixing diverse audiences and diverse usages are still to be considered in educational history, as they are also in nursing history.

One should not stop there, though, for this problem, which is at root one of finding ways to disseminate and popularize special knowledge without oversimplification, is evident in all fields of history. More even, it is a problem evident in all fields of scholarship. The frequent failure of academics to comunicate across the boundaries of their expertise, in order to talk with and learn from other academics, other professionals, and the public at large, has been repeatedly noted. And if that failure reflects, among other things, some of the status-related political problems of professionalism, and is of interest for that reason, it is of even greater interest and more serious concern because it also diminishes the possibilities for wide, meaningful, and informed participation in the public processes of decision making. If in nursing history and through nursing history, divisions between academic historians and practitioners and between both of those groups and larger "publics" can be recognized, discussed, studied, and perhaps even bridged, a large problem, manifested in relatively smaller form, may be addressed, and perhaps more profoundly understood.[9]

These briefly sketched possibilities are most assuredly ambitious dreams, and, while integral to the purposes of this book, should not be confused with its more immediate and more modest goals. By making available a number of new studies, this book seeks, primarily, to demonstrate some of the ways in which the history of nursing is broadening and diversifying. Only in that way does the book seek also to promote consideration of what nursing history has been, is now, and may be in the future. Only in that way is the book directly concerned to bring the still not fully recognized, not sufficiently tapped possibilities of the field into clearer view.

The essays to be found here are not joined by any single theme or model or style. They are joined, rather, by a diversely expressed but common effort to understand and to find ways to understand an important aspect of our past. Thus, in various ways, they explore relationships between nursing, the development of health care services, and the formation and transformation of occupational structures. In addition they examine nursing as an arena in which attitudes and values having to do with gender, ethnicity, and social class have intersected with questions of social status and power in revealing, intriguing, and important ways. By studying these questions and others, they illustrate that nursing history provides a telescope through which to examine some of the perceptions and behaviors that have directly and indirectly defined the culture and the institutions with which we have lived.

Susan Armeny's essay deals with cooperation and conflict between trained nurses and female philanthropists during two periods of military emergency. Equally important, it raises questions concerning the merits of several interpretations of cross-class sororal relationships for elucidating what took place in the politics of American nursing at the beginning of the twentieth century. Celia Davies's essay shares with Armeny's an interest in nursing politics and in cooperative undertakings among nurses and philanthropists, this time among people on both sides of the Atlantic. In contrast to Armeny, however, Davies finds it useful to combine with her discussion of historical personalities and events a concern for developing more precise concepts for looking at the professionalization process itself. Further, whereas Armeny finds cause to suggest modifications in the existing historical interpretations she deals with, Davies finds in a number of often criticized "consensus" views of American character the insight necessary to make sense of the phenomena she has observed.

Jane Pacht Brickman and Karen Buhler-Wilkerson study the development—the stunted development, they argue—of once promising fields of home health services, Brickman focusing on midwifery, Buhler-Wilkerson on public health nursing. Alike in their recognition of the problems encountered in both areas, and in their dismay over those problems, Brickman and Buhler-Wilkerson nevertheless differ in their reading of the various causative factors involved.

The essays by Nancy Tomes and Susan Reverby are noteworthy not only for the historical data they present, concerning, in the first instance, the politics of nurse registration, and, in the second, the decline of private duty nursing, but also for the insights they offer concerning new approaches to these questions of long-standing importance in the field. Tomes, by suggesting the value of thinking of registration as a process rather than as an event, and Reverby, by suggesting the importance of looking at both the alternatives taken and those not taken as hospitals became the predominant setting for nurses' work, have isolated questions that may be used in looking at a variety of "turning points" in nursing's past.

Like Tomes and Reverby, Barbara Melosh also looks at a familiar matter in a fresh way. By drawing on fiction as well as evidence of hospital practices, she explores the ways in which general attitudes toward women have been played out in views of "the nurse" and her role. Like a number of the other essays, therefore, Melosh's study illustrates how new and still relatively unexplored sources of data can link questions about the history of nursing to other questions of even larger moment, in this instance questions having to do with gender-related attitudes and roles. Finally, in the bibliography that closes the book, Mary Ann Dzuback briefly describes and comments upon some recent work in the field.

All the essays have been more or less directly derived from larger studies recently completed or still underway. They have been revised since their initial presentation at the Rockefeller Archive Center Conference, but all are of sufficient interest substantively and methodologically to warrant consideration of where and how they might be still further refined, extended, and applied in future work. Should the essays help to provoke that kind of thinking and talk, the purposes of this book will have been amply achieved.

NOTES

1. An outstanding example of the early emphases of women's history is Eleanor Flexner, *Century of Struggle: The Woman's Rights Movement in the United States*, rev. ed. (Cambridge, Mass.: Harvard University Press, 1975). The changing emphases within the field may be traced through collections such as Mary Hartman and Lois W. Banner, eds., *Clio's Consciousness Raised: New Perspectives on the History of Women* (New York: Harper & Row, 1974) and Berenice A. Carroll, ed., *Liberating Women's History: Theoretical and Critical Essays* (Urbana: University of Illinois Press, 1976); and through historiographical reviews and symposia such as Barbara Sicherman, "Review Essay: American History," *Signs* 1 (1975): 461–85; Gerda Lerner, "Placing Women in History: Definitions and Challenges," *Feminist Studies* 3 (1975): 5–14 (reprinted in *The Majority Finds Its Past: Placing Women in History* [New York: Oxford University Press, 1979]); and Ellen DuBois, Mari Jo Buhle, Temma Kaplan, Gerda Lerner, and Carroll Smith-Rosenberg, "Women's Culture in Women's History: A Symposium," *Feminist Studies* 6 (1980): 26–75. Journals such as *Signs* and *Feminist Studies* are useful indicators of changing trends, as are the papers presented at the various Berkshire Conferences on the History of Women, which have been collected at the Schlesinger Library, Radcliffe College, Cambridge, Massachusetts.

2. Bernard Bailyn, *Education in the Forming of American Society* (Chapel Hill: University of North Carolina Press, 1960); Lawrence A.

Cremin, *The Wonderful World of Ellwood Patterson Cubberley: An Essay on the Historiography of American Education* (New York: Bureau of Publications, Teachers College, Columbia University, 1965); *Traditions of American Education* (New York: Basic Books, 1977), chap. 4; Michael B. Katz, *The Irony of Early School Reform* (Cambridge, Mass.: Harvard University Press, 1968); *Class, Bureaucracy, and Schools: The Illusion of Educational Change in America* (New York: Praeger, 1971); Douglas Sloan, "Historiography and the History of Education," *Review of Research in Education* 1 (1973): 239–69; and Geraldine Jonçich Clifford, "Education: Its History and Historiography," *Review of Research in Education* 4 (1976): 210–67.

    3. Short but incisive reviews of developments in the history of medicine, along with essays representing new directions in the field, may be found in Patricia Branca, ed., *The Medicine Show: Patients, Physicians, and the Perplexities of the Health Revolution in Modern Society* (New York: Science History Publications, 1977), especially Gerald Grob, "The Social History of Medicine and Disease in America: Problems and Possibilities," pp. 1–19; Judith W. Leavitt and Ronald L. Numbers, eds., *Sickness and Health in America: Readings in the History of Medicine and Public Health* (Madison: University of Wisconsin Press, 1978); Susan Reverby and David Rosner, eds., *Health Care in America: Essays in Social History* (Philadelphia: Temple University Press, 1979); Charles Rosenberg, ed., *Healing and History: Essays for George Rosen* (New York: Science History Publications, 1979); and Morris J. Vogel and Charles E. Rosenberg, eds., *The Therapeutic Revolution: Essays in the Social History of American Medicine* (Philadelphia: University of Pennsylvania Press, 1979). The best-known critique of "radical revisionist" work in education is Diane Ravitch, *The Revisionists Revised: A Critique of the Radical Attack on the Schools* (New York: Basic Books, 1977). Similar issues in medical history are presented, albeit in briefer form, in a controversy that appeared in the book review section of the *Bulletin of the History of Medicine* 54 (1980): 131–40, and 589–620.

    4. The works directly revelant to the examples cited here are: Mary O. Furner, *Advocacy and Objectivity: A Crisis in the Professionalization of American Social Science, 1865–1905* (Lexington: The University Press of Kentucky, 1975); Thomas L. Haskell, *The Emergence of Professional Social Science: The American Social Science Association and the Nineteenth-Century Crisis of Authority* (Urbana: University of Illinois Press, 1977); Henrika Kuklick, "The Organization of Social Science in the United States," *American Quarterly* 28 (1976): 124–41; David F. Noble, *America by Design: Science, Technology, and the Rise of Corporate Capitalism* (New York: Oxford University Press, 1977); and Anthony M. Platt, *The Child Savers: The Invention of Delinquency* (Chicago: University of Chicago Press, 1969). However, new work along these lines may be found in monographs as varied as: Jerold S. Auerbach, *Unequal Justice: Lawyers and Social Change in Modern America* (New York: Oxford University Press, 1981); Burton J.

Bledstein, *The Culture of Professionalism: The Middle Class and the Development of Higher Education in America* (New York: W. W. Norton, 1976); Eliot Friedson, *Profession of Medicine: A Study of the Sociology of Applied Knowledge* (New York: Harper & Row, 1970); Carole E. Joffe, *Friendly Intruders: Childcare Professionals and Family Life* (Berkeley: University of California Press, 1977); Paul H. Mattingly, *The Classless Profession: American Schoolmen in the Nineteenth Century* (New York: New York University Press, 1975); Alexandra Oleson and John Voss, eds., *The Organization of Knowledge in Modern America, 1860–1920* (Baltimore: Johns Hopkins University Press, 1979); Charles E. Rosenberg, *No Other Gods: On Science and American Social Thought* (Baltimore: Johns Hopkins University Press, 1976); and Sheila M. Rothman, *Woman's Proper Place: A History of Changing Ideals and Practices, 1870 to the Present* (New York: Basic Books, 1978).

5. For fuller statements of the various definitions of professions suggested above, see Abraham Flexner, "Is Social Work a Profession," *School and Society* 1 (1915): 901–11; Walter P. Metzger, "What Is a Profession?" *Columbia University, Seminar Reports* 3 (1975): 1–12; Magali Sarfatti Larson, *The Rise of Professionalism: A Sociological Analysis* (Berkeley: University of California Press, 1977); and Harold Wilensky, "The Professionalization of Everyone," *American Journal of Sociology* 70 (1964): 137–58. Among the many other discussions of what a profession is, the following are particularly helpful: A. M. Carr-Saunders and P. A. Wilson, *The Professions* (Oxford: Clarendon Press, 1933); Everett C. Hughes, "Professions," *Daedalus* 92 (1963): 655–68; Wilbert E. Moore, with Gerald W. Rosenblum, *The Professions: Roles and Rules* (New York: Russell Sage Foundation, 1970); and Talcott Parsons, "Professions," *International Encyclopedia of the Social Sciences* (New York: Macmillan, 1968). Among the best-known monographs that deal with the importance of professions in "modern" societies are Robert H. Wiebe, *The Search for Order, 1877–1920* (New York: Hill and Wang, 1967) and Daniel Bell, *The Coming of Post-Industrial Society: A Venture in Social Forecasting* (New York: Basic Books, 1973). See also Louis Galambos, "The Emerging Organizational Synthesis in Modern American History," *Business History Review* 44 (1970): 279–90.

6. Amitai Etzioni, ed., *The Semi-Professions and Their Organization: Teachers, Nurses, Social Workers* (New York: Free Press, 1969).

7. The terms "major" and "minor" professions, though not explicitly applied to nursing, are used in Nathan Glazer, "The Schools of the Minor Professions," *Minerva* 12 (1974): 346–64.

8. M. Adelaide Nutting and Lavinia L. Dock, *A History of Nursing: The Evolution of Nursing Systems from the Earliest Times to the Foundation of the First English and American Training Schools for Nurses*, 2 vols. (New York: G. P. Putnam's Sons, 1907). Barbara W. Tuchman, *Practicing History: Selected Essays* (New York: Alfred A. Knopf, 1981) provides useful

insight into some of the stylistic qualities of historical writing with wide general appeal.

9.   Two recent examples of discussions that touch on this point are Carl N. Degler, "Presidential Address: Remaking American History," *Journal of American History* 67 (1980): 7–25 and Gerald Holton, "Where Is Science Taking Us?" The 1981 Jefferson Lectures as reported in *The Chronicle of Higher Education*, May 18, 1981, pp. 3–4.

2

Organized Nurses, Women Philanthropists, and the Intellectual Bases for Cooperation Among Women, 1898–1920

Susan Armeny

On a February morning in 1899 women crowded the opulent home of Washington's leading hostess. There was little to indicate that the gathering of wives of legislators and officials marked the first venture into national politics by organized American nurses. The meeting was chaired first by Lena Potter Cowdin, best known as the daughter of a public-spirited Episcopal bishop, and then by Margaret Chanler, a socialite "whose heroic and valuable services" to sick soldiers in the recent war had "made her name a household one," according to a gushing newspaper account. Only after a leader of the Daughters of the American Revolution, a lobbyist prominent in Republican women's groups, and Chanler spoke did audience demand persuade a few nurses to tell their war "experience." Not nurses but their lay allies explained that the meeting was intended to generate support for a law establishing a permanent body of trained women nurses in the American army.[1]

Another Washington meeting, in August 1918, suggested how organized nurses' efforts to influence federal policies had changed in the intervening nineteen years. A committee of nurses and physicians, representing government and voluntary organizations and civilian interests, met in the office of Dr. Franklin Martin, medicine's spokesman on the Advisory Commission of the wartime Council of National Defense (CND). Only one woman who was not a nurse was present, representing the CND's Woman's Committee. When the participants argued over ways of meeting the demand for women to nurse the troops, nurses spoke for themselves.[2]

The contrasts between the 1899 and 1918 meetings were striking. One was attended by laywomen who were expected to forward nurses' political goals through wifely influence on their husbands, the other by professionals. In the first, leisure-class women spoke for nurses; in the second, nurses made their own case. The two meetings dramatized the rise and decline of a political alliance between organized nurses and leisure-class women. What motivated and enabled women of such dissimilar backgrounds to cooperate? What factors later discouraged such cooperation? Efforts to answer these questions suggest that organized nurses benefited from the tradition of female cooperation and solidarity that had developed among nineteenth-century American women, but that they were not committed to the "social feminism" often associated with that tradition.

Historians have emphasized nineteenth-century women's unprecedented tendency to cooperate with each other in all-female voluntary organizations. The pioneering religious and benevolent groups of the 1810s and 1820s were soon followed by more daring organizations dedicated to reforming society and changing women's position. By the end of the century an abundance of all-female groups offered women chances for companionship, self-development, social service, and collective advancement. One reason for this proliferation of women's groups was the sense of a special female identity created, or at least intensified, by the gap between men's and women's experiences and responsibilities in an increasingly specialized urban and industrial economy. The success of the organizations in turn reinforced women's sense of their special shared identity. The belief that their gender bound women to each other was dramatically evident in the efforts of middle- and upper-class women to know, aid, and learn from poorer women. From antebellum moral reform societies to the settlement houses and Women's Trade Union League of the early twentieth century there were repeated attempts to unite women of different social classes.[3]

Several historians have suggested that efforts to unite women engendered and were sustained by "social feminism." William L. O'Neill, in a pioneering study of American feminism, used the phrase to designate the outlook of early twentieth-century women "who, while believing in women's rights, generally subordinated them to broad social reforms they thought more urgent." J. Stanley Lemons, in a history of women's support for reform in the 1920s, applied this label to the social welfare interests of women's organizations. Although O'Neill and Lemons focused on what social feminists did, they also offered insight into what they believed. O'Neill found social feminism exemplified in organizations that emphasized female solidarity and sought social justice. Lemons asserted that long before Progressivism women's organizations had pursued the social feminist goal of making their "communities more 'homelike.'" A fuller and more explicit analysis of social feminist "consciousness" was provided by Ellen Condliffe Lagemann in a study of five women reformers active at the turn of the century. They believed women's maternal instinct gave them a special "sensitivity to basic human needs" and obligated them to unite in efforts to make American life kinder and more harmonious. All three historians identified social feminism with three related beliefs: that women had a distinctive nature; that it was their nature to be nurturant and altruistic; and that they should therefore band together in order to harmonize and humanize American society, remaking it on the model of an idealized home. All agreed that social feminism had its heyday in the early twentieth century, at the time when organized nurses and women philanthropists made common cause.[4]

How was organized nurses' political alliance with philanthropic women related to the traditions of cooperation among women and the social feminist outlook? The answer is complicated. The alliance was an instance of collaboration among women of different social classes, although neither party cared to emphasize a fact that might damage nurses' pride. Both nurses and philanthropists assumed that they shared special concerns and that these should be promoted by united efforts in which men would play only a marginal part. Decades of organizational activity by women had helped to create these assumptions. The joint political ventures of nurses and laywomen expressed Progressive-era women's interest in public issues that touched on a traditional female responsibility for health care. The ventures thus resembled much of the child welfare movement and parts of the public health movement.[5] However, a close look at the course of the alliance shows that it was not based on shared allegiance to social feminist values and ideas. The participants did not habitually use rhetoric invoking women's distinctive nature, nurturance, and responsibility to humanize society. Their actions indicated that the evils they sought to combat were not the greed, selfishness, and cruelty to the defenseless that troubled social feminists so much as decentralization, disorder, and amateurism. Historians have regarded an impulse to female solidarity as a basic feature in social feminism, and the very existence of the alliance demonstrated this impulse. But there were significant limits to the solidarity the allies manifested. Organized nurses and the laywomen who befriended them were evidently not embarrassed when their political efforts pitted them against other women. Often their women opponents favored systems of nursing compatible with social feminist ideas of women's talents and responsibilities, but incompatible with organized nurses' professional aspirations. Organized nurses' increasing tendency to rely on men as political allies suggests that for them women's solidarity was more an unexamined habit than a consciously cherished ideal. In sum, the alliance between nurses' organizations and philanthropic women rested on an assumption that nurses' goals were of particular concern to other women—presumably because nurses were women fulfilling a traditionally womanly function. But the allies never emphasized women's special nature and role, did not dream of making society homelike, and always hedged their commitment to women's solidarity.

If social feminism did not provide the shared ideas and values that enabled nurses and women philanthropists to cooperate, what did? In an influential study of the United States at the turn of the century, historian Robert Wiebe has argued that in the early twentieth century a "new middle class," with self-conscious professionals in the vanguard, led a "revolution in values" that eventuated in the triumph of "bureaucratic thought." The leaders of organized nurses conformed to Wiebe's model in some ways: they identified strongly with their occupation, devoted themselves to organizing its members, and advocated efficiency and bureaucracy. But their values were not the ones Wiebe described. New middle-class professionals supposedly glorified a "society in indeterminate process" where disinterested bureaucrats presided over "frictionless" organizations smoothly adjusting the claims of "interacting groups." Nurses only rarely revealed their social vision, but when they did they praised expertise, collective purpose, and discipline. Their often unavailing struggles to shape the institutions where nurses worked showed no liking for indeterminate process or an endless tug-of-war between interacting groups. Instead they fought to give nurse executives definite control of their subordinates and autonomy in relation to nonnurse superiors. Since the philanthropic women who backed nurses' efforts were certainly not members of any middle class—new or old—and were quite untouched by formal professional training and work, Wiebe's thesis cannot explain their enthusiastic support of nurses' demands. The alliance between nurses and rich women did not depend on shared adherence to novel bureaucratic values.[6]

This paper argues that the intellectual basis for the alliance was neither social feminism nor bureaucratic thought but an older complex of attitudes, which may be called the Sanitary ideal. Nurses and lay-women active in founding and managing nurses' training schools knew this ideal from the work and writings of Florence Nightingale, but it was first propounded in the United States by the Civil War Sanitary Commission. Upper-class Sanitary leaders, loathing individualism, com-mercialism, and waste, tried to systematize private aid to Union troops and encourage "order and discipline" in army camps and civilian society. Commission spokesmen believed organizations attained efficiency when people specially equipped by birth or training controlled them and when authority flowed downward through a clearly defined hierarchy.[7]

The following narrative will show that in the wake of the Spanish-American War organized nurses and their leisure-class backers strove to establish a war nursing system embodying this concept of efficiency. By 1910 they had a reasonably satisfactory arrangement in the Army Nurse Corps and a reserve provided by nurse enrollment in the Red Cross. When the United States entered World War I that arrangement and the federal government's increasing support for nationally coordi-nated, professionally directed civilian participation in war service re-duced nurses' need for help from philanthropic women and increased the benefits of alliance with medical spokesmen. One World War I epi-sode demonstrated that nurses' organizations could still seek and get im-portant aid from philanthropic women. But the varied support they marshaled in two other wartime emergencies indicated that nurses no longer had to turn to leisure-class women for aid. During World War I nurses benefited from the sense of women's solidarity felt by militant suffragists as well as elite philanthropists. By then nurse leaders generally preferred to rely on political support from physicians and other profes-sionals, thereby emphasizing their identity as professionals over their identity as women. Nurses' new public image, capacity for maneuver, and political alliances did not mean that they had altered their essential goals. During and after the Spanish-American War they had entered the political arena in order to keep war nursing for an elite of well-trained nurses, establish a hierarchy of nurses within army hospitals, and give nurses control and supervision of all nursing work in the hospitals. Dur-ing and after World War I they continued to seek these elusive goals, guided by the Sanitary ideal.

The leaders of nurses' organizations had been instructed in that ideal as training-school pupils. The Sanitary Commission's work directly inspired some of the wealthy laywomen who helped introduce nurses' training schools into the United States in the 1870s. Still more of the founders indicated their concept of good order by borrowing the English Nightingale schools' emphasis on discipline and hierarchy and by hastening to put pupil nurses into uniform. Although some nurses rebelled against the regimentation of training-school life, others embraced it. Training-school superintendents, who had to manage hospital wards staffed by women just learning their trade and to contend with medical superiors who grudged them authority, extolled discipline and claimed that successful hospital nursing depended on giving nurse superintendents plenary power. They told and retold how the first American training school, established in Bellevue Hospital in 1873, had redeemed the hospital by introducing "accurate reports, exact obedience, cleanliness and order." About forty years after the Bellevue school's founding a leading nurse asserted that Bellevue Hospital had been "revolutionized, and so eventually were the other hospitals which one by one adopted the new system. Law, order and decency were established."[8]

In the 1890s training-school superintendents spearheaded the drive to organize two national nurses' groups, the Superintendents' Society and the Nurses' Associated Alumnae. Their leaders assumed that nurses could upgrade their occupation without lay assistance, but the reforms they advocated would have been acceptable to the ladies and gentlemen of the Sanitary Commission. They tried to make training-school curricula more uniform, arrange instruction and ward experience into an educative sequence, and keep women lacking education and refinement out of the schools. Such reforms would have made trained nurses a small, well-trained, homogeneous, self-conscious elite.[9]

Organized nurses' first response to the Spanish-American War showed their confidence that government officials would approve this vision of nursing. Two days after the United States declared war on Spain the Nurses' Associated Alumnae (NAA) met in their first convention. At the suggestion of Isabel Hampton Robb, their president and the great champion of nurses' organizations, the delegates voted to offer their association's services to the government. Robb dispatched a telegram to the secretary of war and went to Washington to reiterate her group's offer. Before the war the United States Army had not employed trained nurses, so it was easy for Robb to "believ[e] that a personal interview, explaining the number and standing of [the NAA] nurses, would result in the acceptance of their services." But Army Surgeon General George Sternberg had already surrendered some one thousand applications from would-be war nurses to an ad hoc Hospital Corps formed by the Daughters of the American Revolution (DAR). From these and later applicants the DAR Hospital Corps chose nurses to be offered army contracts. Individual NAA members did apply and serve as war nurses, but the association itself took no part in the war. Robb regretted the surgeon general's decision, recalling her initial "[v]isions of what splendid systematic work might be done if the nursing might only be in the hands of the nurses themselves." She believed "chaos and confusion" and appointments of "the well-meaning 'born nurse,' the enthusiastic patriot, . . . sisterhoods and . . . adventuresses" resulted from the decision.[10]

Dr. Anita Newcomb McGee, a Washington physician and DAR officer, suggested the Hospital Corps, directed its work, and in September 1898 joined the surgeon general's staff to take charge of army nursing. If nurses' alliances with laywomen had resulted mainly from similar experience of the female condition, nurse leaders would have gravitated toward McGee rather than leisure-class philanthropists. They had much in common. McGee, the daughter of a distinguished astronomer, was born in 1864 and educated in genteel private schools. Although she loved parties and flirtations, a craving for a demanding and purposeful life led her to do anthropological research, study medicine, and plunge into women's club work. Both McGee and her contemporaries among nurse leaders, like Isabel Hampton Robb, grew up at a time when there were few roles for middle-class American women outside the kitchen, parlor, and schoolroom. Driven by unusual energy and ambition, they often made arduous individual searches for alternative roles. These searches led them to idealize professional life as liberating for themselves and other women.[11]

It was an interest in freeing women's energies and harnessing them to social purposes that drew McGee into nursing affairs. She began with the aim of developing a significant volunteer role for DAR women, but soon became enthusiastic about making a permanent place for trained nurses in the American military. By September 1898 she described the army's acceptance of nurses as an event to gladden "womankind in general." Throughout her army service McGee showed a sense of solidarity with other women and a special, if sometimes patronizing "sympathy" with nurses, whom she perceived as her "fellow-professional women."[12]

Nonetheless, McGee's policies alienated nurse leaders. She preferred trained nurses but, having spent her life in official Washington where her father and husband were government scientists, she was ready to bow to political realities. In theory she required that army nurses meet a minimal professional standard: graduation from a training school and endorsement by its superintendent. The DAR Hospital Corps complied with the surgeon general's wishes by choosing nurses from all over the country, a policy that accorded with President William McKinley's desire to use the war effort to overcome sectionalism but diminished chances for participation by NAA members, who were concentrated in the northeast. At times the DAR Corps set aside the requirement that army nurses be training-school graduates. In May the DAR contemplated accepting nuns and untrained black women, presumably ones immune to yellow fever. In July, after outbreaks of yellow fever in the Caribbean and typhoid fever in stateside army camps sharply increased the demand for nurses, the army did employ nuns, black women, and, in a few hospitals hit hard by the typhoid epidemic, women who applied directly to the surgeons in charge. But close to three-fourths of the nurses who signed army contracts between May 1898 and July 1899 were graduates.[13]

Although Robb was mistaken when she implied that McGee did not distinguish between trained and untrained nurses, there was a difference between the kind of army nursing service the NAA favored and the one the DAR set up. The "chaos and confusion" Robb denounced resulted from a heterogeneous nursing force, reflecting the heterogeneity of American society, and from physician McGee's belief that Washington officials must not interfere with army physicians' control over nurses in their particular hospitals. During the summer of 1898 McGee and her DAR comrades simply processed applications, notified nurses when their services were wanted, and sent nurses where army medical officers requested. There the nurses, sometimes without the guidance of a chief nurse, met as best they could the distrust of military physicians and the near universal recalcitrance of enlisted hospital corpsmen. McGee seemed indifferent to organized nurses' desire for hospitals staffed by a homogeneous elite of nurses under the full control of nurse executives.[14]

Other women interested in war work had more sympathy with that ideal. The war's popularity stimulated widespread civilian interest in helping the troops. Upper-class New Yorkers, including Episcopal bishop Henry C. Potter and banker and former vice-president Levi P. Morton, did their bit through the American National Red Cross Relief Committee. Among its numerous women's auxiliaries one eventually "decided to place trained women nurses in the army hospitals." This purpose made the leaders of Auxiliary No. 3 rivals to McGee; their sense of elite social responsibility and experience in hospital and charity work gave them an outlook akin to that of organized nurses.[15]

Three Auxiliary leaders had a decisive impact on relations between women philanthropists and organized nurses. Lena Potter Cowdin, daughter of Bishop Potter and wife of a textile manufacturer, had no previous involvement with medical charity but some experience in civil service reform. Elisabeth Mills Reid had inherited not only her banker father's money but also his interest in endowing and guiding hospitals. She had joined the Board of Managers of the Bellevue Training School for Nurses in 1883 and served until 1931. As the wife of Whitelaw Reid, owner of the *New York Tribune* and spokesman for the Republican party, she had access to national leaders. The third member of the trio was less conspicuous because she disliked "publicity, meetings and promiscuous talk," but her very name connoted influence. Anna Roosevelt Cowles also continued a father's interest in hospitals and had connections with powerful Republicans, through her brother Theodore.[16]

In mid-July 1898 Reid and Cowdin went to Washington to offer Auxiliary-supported nurses for service in stateside army hospitals. Reid later reported that the president "considerately granted the Committee an immediate interview, and very kindly arranged a conference at the White House, with the Secretary of War and the Surgeon-General." Surgeon General Sternberg, until then resistant to Red Cross offers, was soon sending medical officers' requests for nurses directly to Reid. McGee, with Sternberg's backing, tried to preserve her system for employing women nurses in army hospitals. She persuaded Auxiliary leaders to have their nurses "certified by Dr. McGee as conforming to the army standard" and asked them to induce the nurses to sign army contracts and take army pay. Nonetheless the Auxiliary continued to pay some of the nurses it recruited.[17]

The Auxiliary's approach to choosing and placing nurses was more compatible with organized nurses' aspirations than McGee's approach. The DAR system, devised by McGee, let laywomen judge nurses' qualifications, tended to accept all training-school diplomas as equivalent, and treated each nurse as a unit when sending her to work. The Auxiliary's system rested on close cooperation between laywomen and nurse leaders and adherence to Sanitary ideals of elitism and hierarchy. Auxiliary representatives concentrated on fund raising, publicity, and winning official acceptance of nurses. The actual selection of "graduates of good standing, from well-known training schools" was accomplished with "the assistance of the best training-school superintendents in New York." According to a later account, superintendent Anna Maxwell organized an "informal committee" of superintendents who "established correspondence with training-school heads of prominence elsewhere asking them to choose nurses." Unlike McGee, the Auxiliary often sent hospitals graded groups of nurses with a nurse superintendent and sometimes an assistant superintendent already in charge. Isabel Robb believed that it "was through this Auxiliary that the best nursing [in the war] was done."[18]

Leaders of nurses' organizations, having learned their political weakness, wanted to be sure their plans to put army nursing on a permanent basis had "the endorsement of the people at large and especially those who had studied the question." A December 1898 meeting of Robb and other NAA members with Reid, Cowdin, and a woman lawyer provided the desired, if scarcely popular, endorsement and led to formation of a committee to push for legislation establishing a permanent graduate nurse service in the army. All committee members were women. Those who dominated the group's dealings with outsiders were laywomen who had been active in Auxiliary No. 3. Other lay members had participated in founding the Bellevue School a quarter century earlier or in DAR activities. Nurses on the committee had either served under Auxiliary No. 3 sponsorship or been connected with the Johns Hopkins Training School and the movement to organize nurses, both ventures led by Isabel Robb. The one exception was a symbolic figure, Linda Richards, revered as the first nurse to earn an American training-school diploma. Although about half the committee's members were nurses, of the eight women who served as committee officers seven were laywomen.[19]

The division of labor between laywomen and nurses on the committee resembled arrangements in Auxiliary No. 3 during the war: laywomen attended to finance, public relations, and contacts with officialdom; nurses attended to contacts with nurses and physicians and to professional goals. Leisure-class women presented the committee's case to a House of Representatives committee in February 1899 and must have arranged the gathering of office-holders' wives held with such fanfare the same day. They visited officials and legislators to seek counsel and support, usually unaccompanied by nurses. Nurses sought and got endorsements for their bill from the nurses' groups, prominent physicians, and the American Medical Association. According to nurse Anna Maxwell the committee entrusted actual drafting of the first bill it backed to nurses representing the two national associations. Whoever did draft the bill designed it to harmonize with the program for training-school reform espoused by the Superintendents' Society and Associated Alumnae. While lay people and doctors told general audiences that the bill would promote the uncontroversial goal of good nursing for sick and wounded soldiers, it was nurses who justified the bill's specific, controversial provisions to other members of their guild.[20]

At their first meeting Robb won Reid and Cowdin's assent to the nurse leaders' program: "The Nursing Department of the Army should be as thoroughly organized as any other department . . . and managed entirely by nurses." Details of successive bills that the committee backed showed that thorough organization meant a hierarchy of nurses, all boasting the best professional training then available. The bill introduced in January 1899 provided for a nurse at the head of the army nursing service, four grades of nurses below her, and a nursing service commission. The office of the superintendent was to be lofty, since she was appointed by the president and confirmed by the Senate, and lucrative, since she was paid more than leading training-school superintendents or Dr. McGee. All army nurses had to possess the two-year general hospital training necessary for membership in the NAA. The nursing service commission—composed of the secretary of war, high army officers, a laywoman, and two civilian nurses—would nominate candidates for superintendent, approve the rules she made, and pass on credentials of would-be army nurses.[21]

Two goals were paramount: attracting into army nursing "women of the higher type," "the right kind of women," and replacing Dr. McGee with a nurse. In February 1899 committee members intimated that they were ready to compromise on some features of the bill, but would "stand firmly by the provision that the superintendent of nurses shall be a trained nurse." The nursing service commission was apparently intended to give representatives of civilian-trained nurses and their supporters among laywomen power to install a like-minded superintendent and to ensure selection of the right kind of nurses. These purposes emerged more clearly when the committee briefly proposed an all-woman commission, with no ex-officio members and with a nurse majority.[22]

This ambitious measure got a surprisingly friendly reception from members of the House Military Affairs Committee, who unanimously reported it out, and from the whole House. Many of the representatives were for the moment disgusted with the Army Medical Department's wartime performance and were willing to tinker with its organization. The following year a more moderate version, put forward to meet objections from the surgeon general and McGee, fared poorly, dying in committee in both houses. In the spring of 1900 Bill Committee members pared down their requests to the "principles" they deemed "vital": a permanent, all-graduate nursing service and a graduate nurse with general hospital training as superintendent. That fall the surgeon general asked McGee to draft a section on nurses for an army reorganization bill designed to adjust the army to the new demands of empire. Her draft provided for a graduate nurse force headed by a superintendent with no defined qualifications. The Senate Military Affairs Committee amended her plan to give nurses the prize they desired, a trained nurse, graduated from a two-year course, as superintendent.[23]

The Bill Committee's formula for good nursing—centralized authority, hierarchy, and elite recruitment—had limited appeal to legislators or officials but strong support from private citizens actively interested in army nursing. Even the committee's arch-foe, McGee, wanted a unified force of trained, graduate nurses. When she did champion values inconsistent with the Sanitary ideal—like equal opportunity for graduates of small and obscure training schools—only unorganized individuals applauded. The organized groups, male, female, lay, and professional, all sided with the committee. Although the DAR owed its role in army nursing to McGee, an officer of that group proclaimed "that the Daughters of the Revolution, who had stood by the trained nurses during the last summer, cordially supported this bill now." Many Americans favored local decentralized recruitment of nurses and employment of amateurs or those with nursing experience but no formal training. The thousands of laywomen who volunteered in the spring of 1898 and the Chicago women physicians and nurses who assured McGee of their "unanimous . . . wish to serve our Illinois troops; [because] we feel that this will assuage the grief and suspense of the Illinois women in the home" were among them. But in the postwar debate over army nursing virtually no one defended amateurs and local recruitment.[24]

The committee hailed establishment of a nurse-led Army Nurse Corps (ANC) as victory, but the corps at first fell short of committee hopes. As a result of the resistance from McGee, the surgeon general, and legislators swayed by these officials' judgment, the corps was neither as elite in its membership, nor as clearly under the control of nurses, nor as integrated into the movement to upgrade nursing as they wished. Nurse leaders were better able to bring the ANC into line with their aspirations after 1909 when two of their number served in succession as superintendent. An earlier takeover of the Red Cross by upper-class men and women with a passion for centralized administration and business-like record-keeping had stimulated cooperation between the relief organization and nurses' groups. Nurses were familiar with some of those who reorganized the Red Cross, notably Anna Roosevelt Cowles and Elisabeth Mills Reid. Mabel T. Boardman, who dominated the Red Cross from reorganization until American involvement in World War I, described the Sanitary Commission as the true "precursor" of the revitalized Red Cross. The Associated Alumnae welcomed the new outlook at Red Cross headquarters and made suggestions that led to the establishment of a Red Cross Nursing Service composed of training-school graduates who, in wartime, would form a reserve for the Army and Navy Nurse Corps. A committee with a nurse majority guided the service. In 1909, when it began work, the committee's fifteen members included four veterans of the Bill Committee, among them Robb and Reid.[25]

In the years between the Spanish-American War and World War I some developments encouraged ties between nurses and leisure-class women, but most led nurses to look elsewhere for political allies. Nurses heading the growing number of nongovernment public health nursing agencies worked closely with boards of lay managers, composed largely of well-to-do women. A group of such laywomen launched the first successful national magazine on public health nursing, and when public health nurses formed a national organization in 1912 they took the unprecedented step of admitting lay people to a limited membership. However, in efforts to win state nurse registration laws, which were modeled on physicians' license laws, nurses relied most heavily on medical groups and prestigious doctors for aid. Changes in the relationship between the government and occupational interest groups also induced organized nurses to identify with other professionals rather than with laywomen. Woodrow Wilson's administration encouraged occupational groups to join in the war effort by establishing the Advisory Commission of the Council of National Defense, composed of representatives of transportation, education, engineering, finance, commerce, labor, and medicine. President Wilson himself hailed the Advisory Commission as "mark[ing] the entrance of the nonpartisan engineer and professional man into American governmental affairs on a wider scale than ever before . . . efficiency being their sole object and Americanism their only motive."[26]

During World War I organized nurses depended less on their alliance with leisure-class women than at the turn of the century because of the changed setting, their ties with other professionals, and the variety of lay people willing to lend them political support. Even when they turned to philanthropic allies they brought more resources of their own to the partnership than in 1899. Nurse leaders' increased political experience and participation in a network of officially sanctioned interest groups did not promote militancy. While they pursued goals dear to the 1899 Bill Committee and consistent with the Sanitary ideal—especially a monopoly of war nursing by fully trained professionals and establishment of clear-cut, nurse-dominated hierarchies in military hospitals—they were quicker to compromise than their predecessors. Three World War I episodes illuminate organized nurses' complex and uneven movement away from their old alliance with rich women and toward a cautious preoccupation with maintaining professional gains.

Public health nurses, although accustomed to joint effort and even comradeship with leisure-class women, in their first World War I emergency looked to the new Council of National Defense network for aid. Soon after American entry into the war the National Committee on Red Cross Nursing Service, dominated by nurses in other specialties and perhaps complaisant to lay Red Cross leaders, decided against "recognition of public health nursing as a patriotic service equivalent to military duty." As a result the Red Cross could call up public health nurses for military service and disrupt the civilian agencies where they worked. The National Organization for Public Health Nursing (NOPHN) asked a male public health leader who served on its Advisory Council to request addition of a nurse to the CND Advisory Commission. The group sent two nurses to Washington to ask Dr. Franklin Martin, chairman of the CND's General Medical Board (GMB), for a pronouncement on the value of public health nurses' "home service." Although no nurse was invited to join the seven men on the Advisory Commission, a Sub-Committee on Public Health Nursing was grafted to the GMB. This official recognition helped persuade the Red Cross to reverse its decision and sanction civilian service by public health nurses.[27]

Other nurses sought and got CND help in shielding nursing schools and hospitals from pressure to turn out quickly and haphazardly trained nurses. Before the United States declared war Adelaide Nutting, the leading figure in American nursing education, summoned four other nurses to her apartment to discuss the looming threats to nursing education: training schools might suffer as their graduate staffs were drawn into war nursing; untrained college women eager for war service might get to Europe and begin nursing. She proposed that college women be recruited into the training schools, thus deflecting them from amateur nursing, increasing the future supply of nurses, providing ideal substitutes for the teachers, executives, and public health nurses siphoned off, and bringing a valuable elite into the profession. By June 1917 the knot of friends in Nutting's apartment had grown into an elaborate committee that united presidents of the three national nurses' associations, the top-ranking Red Cross nurse, prominent physicians and hospital administrators, and public health leaders—but included no lay philanthropists. The committee energetically promoted nursing as a career for college women and began a census of the nation's nurses designed to show that war needs could be met without recourse to untrained or partly trained nurses. It became part of the CND system on the initiative of the already affiliated Sub-Committee on Public Health Nursing and of Dr. William Welch, a leading spokesman for medicine, old friend of Nutting's, and member of her committee. The GMB and other CND bodies generally backed stands taken by Nutting's committee, even when this caused friction with the War Department or the Red Cross.[28]

Sometimes such backing was not enough. In 1918 nurses agitated for an Army School of Nursing as an alternative to plans for staffing military hospitals with "aids" who had taken brief Red Cross courses and worked a meager month in hospital wards. Trained nurses did not want aids bungling military nursing or competing for postwar nursing jobs armored with the prestige their war service would confer. The CND committee that Nutting chaired had tried to quiet the demand for such sub-nurses by accelerating the preparation of fully trained nurses. Nonetheless, the Red Cross, with the approval of the nurses' organizations, had been training aids. Pressures to use aids mounted in early 1918 as the Allies clamored for American troops and the military speeded up their departure for France. A subordinate warned Secretary of War Newton Baker that the growing army could be adequately nursed only by aids and charged that Nutting's committee was blocking their use. When Baker asked it for advice the Surgeon General's Office prepared to announce that it would hire and pay aids to work in base hospitals. The proposal to pay aids, and the civilian hospital administrators' enthusiasm for the aids plan, raised nurses' fear that the postwar nursing market would be flooded with a new category of low-grade nurses.[29]

Annie W. Goodrich, one of the four nurses called to Nutting's apartment, had just joined the surgeon general's staff as inspector of military hospitals. Flying into action, she sought help from a physician member of Nutting's committee who then worked for the surgeon general, "begging that the Red Cross be asked to withhold this announcement" until she toured base hospitals. The best civilian hospitals were staffed by nurses in training with a few graduates supervising and teaching them. Since the Spanish-American War the larger army hospitals had been staffed by hospital corpsmen with the graduate nurses of the ANC supervising them. Why not staff army hospitals with nurses in training, thereby banishing the corpsmen, who lacked the "desire to excel," and averting employment of aids? Goodrich's determination to exclude aids led her to argue that nurses in training would give better service than even an all-graduate force. She thus undermined justifications for giving professionals thorough training and for the moment forgot how she and Nutting had attacked use of nurse students to staff hospitals as exploitation rather than education.[30]

Despite these ironies Goodrich's plan appealed to the professional-minded. The Surgeon General's Office canceled the call for aids and the Army School proposal won acceptance from a War Department group, nurse members of Nutting's committee, and the surgeon general. While the General Staff pondered the plan, nurses attending the joint annual convention of their three national organizations heard an impassioned plea for aids from Jane Delano, the top-ranking Red Cross nurse, and a rejoinder from Goodrich. They endorsed the Army School plan. When the General Staff vetoed the Army School plan, nurse leaders delegated Goodrich and two laywomen from the board of Cleveland's public health nursing agency to intercede with Secretary of War Baker. The trio succeeded in getting him to authorize establishing an Army School of Nursing.[31]

Their venture showed that alliances between organized nurses and women philanthropists had changed. During the Spanish-American War the women of Auxiliary No. 3 had initiated their own nursing project. The postwar Bill Committee had been a jointly planned effort, in which laywomen outshone nurses. The laywomen brought into the alliance money, access to publicity, and contacts with the mighty. Nurse leaders, who had no comparable resources, tended to exaggerate their allies' political strength. One told another in 1901 that "these [philanthropic] women can . . . do more in a minute than we can in a lifetime." In 1918 nurses appeared more confident, wealthy laywomen more diffident. Nurses launched the Army School plan, promoted it with the help of professional allies, and decided when to bring in lay reinforcements. Frances Payne Bolton, one of the laywomen who accompanied Goodrich to the Secretary of War, was heir to a Standard Oil fortune and a practiced advocate of nurses' interests. She and the third committee member had learned about nursing when the Cleveland debutantes of their year trudged through the slums helping the visiting nurses. At twenty-two, as a new hospital board member, Bolton fought for better housing for nurses in training. She was in 1918 an active member of the NOPHN Advisory Council. She had already tried to shore up nurse training standards by urging young women of her own class to resist temptations to use aid training as "a short cut to nursing."[32]

Despite her background, wealth, and experience in philanthropy, Bolton sounded envious of nurses' competence and usefulness. She told the 1918 nurses' convention that leisure-class women would welcome establishment of the Army School: "We want training and we have felt the need of it more keenly . . . than you can possibly know." Many of her peers might go "into the profession of nursing with . . . thankful spirits that we have been given something of which we have been deprived." Bolton's avowed yearning for training would surely have been incomprehensible to Reid, Cowdin, or Cowles. Sanitary Commission leaders' idea that training, like birth and breeding, justified leadership was giving way to the idea that only training could justify leadership.[33]

Nonetheless, certain features of the alliance between organized nurses and philanthropic women persisted. Like the Auxiliary leaders, Bolton and her companion were volunteers who opposed official acceptance of any but trained professional nurses. They could comfortably attack amateur work at the bedside because wealth and social eminence gave them access to amateur work directing and financing organizations. Both sets of philanthropic women aided nurses in battles waged against other women: in 1899 and 1900 Dr. McGee and nurses who did not meet the professional organizations' standards; in 1918 Jane Delano of the Red Cross and would-be aids. Clearly, what united organized nurses and leisure-class women was not devotion to the interests of women in general but devotion to the interests of women who were bearers of the Sanitary ideal of trained, disciplined service.

Nurses used their ties to medical professionals to join the CND network and maneuver it to serve their goals. They used, first, professional and then philanthropic allies to persuade officials to set up an Army School of Nursing. In their longest and most ambitious World War I era political effort, designed to get army and navy nurses military rank, nurses turned to medical and philanthropic allies only after another group of outsiders had helped to launch the campaign. The outsiders were laywomen, apparently motivated by a sense of solidarity with women in nursing, but members of the militant wing of the cresting suffrage movement rather than the philanthropists who had assisted nurses in other political battles. The struggle for rank thus resulted from two factors: the experience of over twenty thousand civilian nurses who poured into the four-hundred-member ANC and an initiative by some suffragists. Many of the civilian recruits found the position of army nurses a "regular serfdom." Like army nurses from 1898 on, they complained about medical officers' disdain for nurses and, even more, about hospital corpsmen's refusal to follow nurses' directions. Within a month of United States entry into the war organized nurses responded to complaints from their sisters in uniform with a discreet resolution asking for an increase in army nurses' authority.[34]

Militant suffragists connected with the Woman's party soon went further. New Yorkers, led by Harriot Stanton Blatch and wealthy militant Louisine W. Havemeyer, in summer 1917 formed a committee to seek rank for nurses. By then the Woman's party pickets who had ringed the White House since January were being arrested and jailed. Blatch, although a party member, remained aloof from the picket campaign in order to work for the wartime Food Administration. Perhaps she seized on the rank issue because it enabled her to appear simultaneously patriotic, militantly feminist, and sensitive to the needs of working women, a group she had tried to draw into the suffrage movement. Helen Hoy Greeley, a lawyer and political associate of Blatch's, became the group's counsel. The all-woman committee had contacts with a group of New York nurses led by Anna Maxwell, not a suffragist but a veteran of the campaign for an army nursing bill. Behind the scenes Adelaide Nutting complained to Dr. Franklin Martin of the CND about military nurses' conflicts with refractory corpsmen and recommended to the secretary of war rank for nurses.[35]

Advocates of rank for nurses launched a major offensive in the spring of 1918. Two bills seeking rank were introduced in Congress, women's organizations announced support for rank, sympathizers publicized the cause, and both the staid *New York Times* and the executive committee of the CND General Medicine Board gave endorsement.[36]

Although the publicity-conscious Blatch and her suffragist associates had done much to arouse interest in the rank issue, a hearing before the House Military Affairs Committee was dominated by nurses and physicians connected with the war effort. The only laywomen who spoke were Blatch, a lone leisure-class survivor of the bill campaign, and social worker Julia Lathrop, who as a member of Nutting's CND committee might be regarded as representing nurses' views. Suffragist involvement in the campaign for rank had already peaked. Blatch and most of those who had followed her into the campaign ceased to be prominent in it after the 1918 hearings. Their apparent loss of interest coincided with a decision to push only for relative rank. Such rank, Greeley explained to the lawmakers in April 1918, would give nurses the title of officers, their insignia, and the power to command in matters pertaining to their professional responsibility, but not the commissions, pay, or benefits of other officers. Within a month of the hearing the three national nurses' groups announced their support for relative rank.[37]

Visible leadership in the struggle for rank now fell to representatives of organized nurses and to Greeley. In May 1918 a committee representing each of the three national nurses' groups was formed to "work with Mrs. Greeley," and the CND Committee on Nursing, chaired by Nutting, assumed part of the responsibility for her salary. Greeley, although now a paid lobbyist and publicist, was no mere hireling. She cared enough about rank to donate her services for eight weeks and defer seeking pay when funds ran low. She helped to make policy and at times filled arguments for rank with fervid denunciations of male indifference to nurses' rights. Greeley, rather than a nurse with military experience, was brought in to tell the CND General Medical Board that rank was a prerequisite for efficient nursing. Greeley, not a nurse, advised a 1919 nurses' convention to disregard the opinions of some army nurses who disclaimed interest in rank—and, presumably, to listen to her instead. Such reliance on an outsider galled at least one nurse. Sophia Palmer, editor of the *American Journal of Nursing*, privately predicted that "Mrs. Greeley will never get it across" and that rank would not be won until nurses had "someone of our own people in charge of" the campaign. Palmer was wrong. The campaign succeeded in June 1920 when an amendment to an army reorganization bill gave nurses relative rank. Still, Greeley's role raised the question of whether nurses, who had once relied on leisure-class ladies to defend their interests, were now surrendering that task to another kind of outsider, the paid lobbyist.[38]

Why did nurses fight for relative rank, which failed to give them the status, pay, and perquisites of officers? One answer is that they had learned that officials and congressmen would not concede nurses' full claims to be treated as professionals and sought what they might realistically get. The nurses' own standard public answer to this question was a different one, which showed their continuing devotion to concepts of order and efficiency derived from the Sanitary ideal. This answer was well formulated by Jane Delano, a former superintendent of the Army Nurse Corps, in spring 1918.

> Efficient organization in any hospital, civilian or military, is . . . to be secured only by placing definite responsibility upon one person in the ward. . . . [In military hospitals] We have the corps men, we have even the officers themselves, and perhaps the nurses, with the traditions of divided responsibility, and we have this . . . Hospital Corps man, who in the past has not been placed definitely under the nurse.

Capitalizing on the fad for Taylorite efficiency engineering, nurses argued that rank was an efficiency measure and insisted that they were not demanding equality. They sought only protection from the caprices of medical superiors and control over insubordinate hospital corpsmen. Like their predecessors in 1898, they believed efficiency would result from a clear-cut hierarchy with people like themselves in high position. Despite the timely label, their concept of efficiency owed less to the ascendant scientific management movement than to the Sanitary ideal.[39]

Although organized nurses' essential goals had not altered, their ways of pursuing them had. There were dramatic changes in nurses' relations with lay sympathizers. In the turn-of-the-century effort to establish an army nursing service, leisure-class women had been nurses' only important lay allies. In the World War I fight for rank, nurses collected diverse lay supporters. Militant suffragists helped kick off the rank campaign, but—with the exception of Greeley, herself a professional woman—they drifted away long before victory was won. The rank campaigners sought to keep up ties with nurses' leisure-class allies and financial backers by putting rich women from at least five cities on their national committee. But Greeley was soon lamenting that the committee was not "alive and interested." The problem may have been poor choice of members or the decline of lay interest in nurses once the war was over. But perhaps the increasing independence and political savvy of nurse leaders undercut wealthy women's interest in aiding nurses. Some long-time philanthropic allies stayed loyal: Bolton and a New Yorker from the Bellevue training-school board gave generously to the rank campaign without actively participating. Although the money was welcome it is clear that no philanthropic individual or group played a key role in the rank campaign, as Reid had in the agitation for an army nursing service, or Bolton in the fight for the Army School of Nursing.[40]

For the first time nurses deliberately sought political backing from laymen as well as women. When committees were established in each state to mobilize public support for rank, leaders of the national effort suggested to state nurses' groups that "the chairman preferably [should] be a lay person, either a man or a woman." For their national committee nurses secured the weighty influence of conservative former president William Howard Taft, who became honorary chairman.[41]

In the campaign for rank, more than in any of their earlier national political ventures, nurses dominated, both behind the scenes and in public. The diversity of their lay supporters—from feminist Blatch to elder statesman Taft—made them more independent of any one source of support. Nurses were also readier to do their own politicking than in 1899. Joint lay-nurse committees in every state sponsored letter-writing efforts and a congressman paid tribute to the letters sent by nurses with war service. Nurses were the star witnesses at congressional hearings and became experts at button-holing legislators. Nurses' groups gave money to the campaign and a nurse headed its finance committee.[42]

Nurse organizations' decreasing reliance on lay allies, particularly philanthropic women, did not imply increasing militancy, as a compari-

son of earlier and later political campaigns shows. The 1899 bill campaigners, overestimating the political clout of their lay members, at first
demanded utopian measures and only slowly compromised. The better-
backed and more politically experienced 1918 rank campaigners made
their crucial decision to seek only relative rank early in their effort.
Nurses' groups thus used unprecedented, aggressive, and public tactics
in their quest for the modest, seemingly "realistic" goal of relative rank.
(In fact, their modesty did not placate the secretary of war and two successive surgeons general, who fought proposals for any kind of rank.)[43]
The demise of nurse organizations' political alliance with leisure-class
women brought losses as well as gains to nurses.

The alliance between nurses and philanthropic women, which flourished in the first two decades of the twentieth century, illuminates
the relation between nursing history and women's history in several
ways. Women philanthropists' assistance to nurses illustrates the way
Progressive-era women's entry into the political process was precipitated
by issues that had special resonance because they touched on women's
new opportunities and their already sanctioned duties. The arguments
nurses used and the friends they found show how lastingly and profoundly the professional nurse elite were influenced by concepts of social
service espoused by some women volunteers in the mid-nineteenth
century.

Finally, and most significantly, the alliance suggests questions about
the outlook of the many women who sought more active participation
in public life in the Progressive era. We have seen that the ideas and
values of nurses and their philanthropic allies cannot be identified with
either of two outlooks supposedly current in that era—the bureaucratic
faith in indeterminate process and mutual adjustment of group conflicts
as a source of social harmony, and the social feminist vision of a society
made homelike under the guidance of women's maternal instinct. There
is some doubt about whether or not any substantial number of Americans were drawn to the colorless theorems of bureaucratic thought.
There is no doubt that many were drawn to social feminism, which
affirmed the experiences and responsibilities that set women apart from
men while endorsing women's demands for new opportunities. Nurses'
associations, like many other women's groups of their time, occasionally
pulsed with social feminist tendencies, but their cooperation with
wealthy women owed less to social feminism than to mutual allegiance
to the older and harsher precepts of the Sanitary ideal.

One element associated with social feminism was important to that
cooperation—a sense of women's solidarity in good works. Rich women

like Reid and Bolton struggled for the advance of nurses and nursing, accepting the debatable definition of good nursing propounded by the leaders of professional organizations. Still more surprisingly, in 1899, when nurses appeared to be junior partners in the alliance, the women of Auxiliary No. 3 deferred to nurse leaders' opinions. Until the rank campaign, nurses turned to women, not men, when they needed political help from the laity. A sense of an established, comfortable community of women helps to explain these facts. But whatever gender-loyalty nurses and women philanthropists felt did not keep them from battling other women, like Dr. McGee, who had at least equal devotion to the community of women, or from denying that the mere employment of women with their talent for caring would necessarily lead to good nursing.

This study indicates the need for more investigation of the ways an impulse to female solidarity, apart from social feminism, affected women's organizations and their politics. Until now historians have usually examined the sense of women's solidarity when it contributed to reform and feminist movements. But in the early twentieth-century United States that sense was widely diffused and compatible with diverse ideas of a good society. The wide diffusion gave nurses a ready-made constituency, symbolized by the well-to-do women assembled in their behalf in February 1899. The diverse interpretations meant that leaders of nurses' organizations and the philanthropic women who befriended them saw little incompatibility between the military styles of organization they admired and womanliness (unlike many of their reformer contemporaries who linked their sense of women's solidarity to pacifism). We shall not know the varied implications of women's feeling of kinship with each other until there are more studies of the myriad formal and informal groups of Progressive-era women. This account of one improbable association is offered as a contribution toward our understanding of those American women in an age of reform who were not strongly committed to reform, feminism, or social feminism, yet were not content with domesticity and political passivity.

NOTES

References from the American Nurses' Association Records, Nursing History Archives, and Minutes of 18th Annual Convention are reprinted by permission of the American Nurses' Association (ANA).

1. Quotations from "Women as Army Nurses," *New York Tribune*, Feb. 4, 1899, p. 7; cf. "Trained Nurses in the Army," *Washington Post*,

Feb. 4, 1899, p. 7. The hostess is identified in "Mrs. M'Lean Dies After Death Race," *New York Times*, Sept. 10, 1912, p. 11, as the wife of the *Washington Post*'s owner. On participants, see "Mrs. Cowdin's Death," *New York Times*, Oct. 20, 1906, p. 9; *American National Red Cross Relief Committee Reports; May, 1898–March,* 1899 (New York: Knickerbocker Press, n.d.), pp. 262–67 (hereafter cited as *Relief Committee Reports*); and Lavinia L. Dock et al., *History of American Red Cross Nursing* (New York: Macmillan Co., 1922), pp. 48, 67–68, 70 (hereafter cited as Dock, *Red Cross*).

2. U.S. Congress, Senate, *Digest of the Proceedings of the Council of National Defense During the World War: Prepared in Narrative Form by Dr. Franklin H. Martin,* S. Doc. 193, 73rd Cong, 2nd Sess. (Washington, D.C.: Government Printing Office, 1934), pp. 478–79 (hereafter cited as Martin, *Digest*).

3. Nancy F. Cott, *The Bonds of Womanhood: "Woman's Sphere" in New England, 1780–1835* (New Haven: Yale University Press, 1977), esp. pp. 149–57; Barbara J. Berg, *The Remembered Gate: Origins of American Feminism: The Woman and the City, 1800–1860* (New York: Oxford University Press, 1978), esp. pp. 198–222; Karen J. Blair, *The Clubwoman as Feminist: True Womanhood Redefined, 1868–1914,* with a preface by Annette K. Baxter (New York: Holmes & Meier, 1980); Nancy Schrom Dye, *As Equals and As Sisters: Feminism, the Labor Movement, and the Women's Trade Union League of New York* (Columbia: University of Missouri Press, 1980).

4. William L. O'Neill, *Everyone Was Brave: A History of Feminism in America,* with a new afterword by the author (New York: Quadrangle, 1971), pp. x, 77–106; J. Stanley Lemons, *The Woman Citizen: Social Feminism in the 1920s* (Urbana: University of Illinois Press, 1973), quotation p. 234; Ellen Condliffe Lagemann, *A Generation of Women: Education in the Lives of Progressive Reformers* (Cambridge, Mass.: Harvard University Press, 1979), pp. 154–59, quotation p. 155. Good examples of the social feminist vision are Jane Addams, *Democracy and Social Ethics,* ed. Anne Firor Scott (Cambridge, Mass.: Belknap Press of Harvard University Press, 1964); Jane Addams, *The Long Road of Woman's Memory* (New York: Macmillan Co., 1916).

5. See, for example, James Johnson, "The Role of Women in the Founding of the United States Children's Bureau," in Carol V. R. George, ed., *"Remember The Ladies:" New Perspectives on Women in American History* (Syracuse: Syracuse University Press, 1975), pp. 179–96.

6. Robert H. Wiebe, *The Search for Order: 1877–1920* (New York: Hill & Wang, 1967), pp. 111–63, quotations pp. 111, 133, 161, 163. There is some evidence that, like nurses, early twentieth-century leaders in certain other professions promoted efficiency essentially as a way of increasing their own power and, like nurses, did *not* cherish the outlook Wiebe attributes to the new middle class. See Wayne K. Hobson, "Professionals, Progressives

and Bureaucratization: A Reassessment," *Historian* 39 (August 1977): 639–58. For glimpses of nurses' aspirations for the larger society, see Mary Adelaide Nutting, *A Sound Economic Basis for Schools of Nursing, and Other Addresses* (New York: G. P. Putnam's Sons, 1926), pp. 105–11, 350–64 (hereafter cited as Nutting, *Economic Basis*); and Annie Warburton Goodrich, *The Social and Ethical Significance of Nursing: A Series of Addresses* (New York: Macmillan Co., 1932) (hereafter cited as Goodrich, *Significance*).

7. George M. Frederickson, *The Inner Civil War: Northern Intellectuals and the Crisis of the Union* (New York: Harper & Row, 1965), esp. pp. 99–112, quotation p. 104; William Quentin Maxwell, *Lincoln's Fifth Wheel: The Political History of the United States Sanitary Commission*, with a preface by Allan Nevins (New York: Longmans, Green & Co., 1956), pp. 10, 15–18.

8. The influence on training schools of martial ideals derived from the Sanitary Commission or from Nightingale is described in M. Adelaide Nutting and Lavinia L. Dock, *A History of Nursing*, 4 vols. (New York: G. P. Putnam's Sons, 1907–12), 2:370–88, 400–402 (hereafter cited as Nutting and Dock, *History*); Anne L. Austin, *The Woolsey Sisters of New York: A Family's Involvement in the Civil War and a New Profession (1860–1900)* (Philadelphia: American Philosophical Society, 1971), pp. 134–38, 151–55; James H. Rodabaugh and Mary Jane Rodabaugh, *Nursing in Ohio: A History* (Columbus: Ohio State Nurses' Association, 1951), p. 65; Sara E. Parsons, *History of the Massachusetts General Hospital Training School for Nurses* (Boston: Whitcomb & Barrows, 1922), pp. 51, 60. The phrases describing the Bellevue school's significance are quoted from Louise Darche, "Proper Organization of Training Schools in America," in Isabel A. Hampton et al., *Nursing of the Sick—1893: Papers and Discussions from the International Congress of Charities, Correction and Philanthropy, Chicago, 1893* (New York: McGraw-Hill Book Co., 1949), p. 93; and M. A. Nutting, "The Work of the Johns Hopkins School for Nurses," *Johns Hopkins Hospital Bulletin* 25 (December 1914): 359. Cf. Linda Richards, "Thirty Years of Progress," *American Journal of Nursing* (hereafter cited as *AJN*) 4 (January 1904): 264; and LLD[ock], "The General Hospital in Vienna," *AJN* 5 (February 1905): 320–23.

9. The American Society of Superintendents of Training Schools for Nurses, commonly called the Superintendents' Society, was founded in 1893 and eventually became the National League of Nursing Education. The Associated Alumnae of Trained Nurses of the United States and Canada was founded in 1897 and eventually became the American Nurses' Association. Although before that transformation the organization's name varied slightly it was often simply called the Associated Alumnae. See Lyndia Flanagan, comp., *One Strong Voice: The Story of the American Nurses' Association* (Kansas City, Mo.: American Nurses' Association, 1976), pp.

23–40 (hereafter cited as Flanagan, *Voice*). The early phases of the campaign to reform training schools are best followed in the *Reports of the Annual Conventions of the American Society of Superintendents of Training Schools for Nurses* (Harrisburg, Pa.: Harrisburg Publishing Co., 1897–   ) (hereafter cited as SS with date). See also Nutting and Dock, *History*, 3:121–41; Isabel Hampton Robb, *Educational Standards for Nurses, With Other Addresses on Nursing Subjects* (Cleveland, Ohio: E. C. Koeckert, 1907) (hereafter cited as Robb, *Educational Standards*). The resistance of hospital administrators, who treated nurses in training as workers rather than students; the limited power of training-school superintendents, who were hospital employees themselves; and disagreements among nurses kept organization leaders from creating the kind of schools and profession they advocated.

10.   The quotations are from an 1899 speech by Isabel Hampton Robb, "Some of the Lessons of the Late War and Their Bearing Upon Trained Nursing," in Robb, *Educational Standards*, pp. 150, 151, 152 (hereafter cited as Robb, "Lessons"). Anita Newcomb McGee, "The Co–Relation of Nurses' Organizations and Army Nursing," *Trained Nurse and Hospital Review* (hereafter cited as TN) 23 (November 1899): 294–97, explained that the NAA telegram arrived in garbled form and charged that Robb expected the government to employ only NAA members. Robb denied the charge that she sought an NAA monopoly, "Lessons," p. 151. "Report of Convention," *TN* 20 (June 1898): 330; Martha L. Sternberg, *George Miller Sternberg: A Biography* (Chicago: American Medical Association, 1920), p. 168, quoting the surgeon general's official report; Anita Newcomb McGee, "Women Nurses in the American Army," *Woman's Medical Journal* (hereafter cited as WMJ) 10 (February 1900): 47; Dita H. Kinney, "Dr. Anita Newcomb McGee and What She Has Done for the Nursing Profession," *TN* 26 (March 1901): 131, quoting June 1898 report to DAR by McGee.

11.   *Notable American Women*, s.v. "McGee, Anita Newcomb," by Mary R. Dearing (hereafter cited as NAW); McGee, "Woman's Work" [1890s] and MS "Idea Book" [1890s], both in Anita Newcomb McGee Papers, Library of Congress, Washington, D.C. Cf. Janet Wilson James, "Isabel Hampton and the Professionalization of Nursing in the 1890s," in *The Therapeutic Revolution: Essays in the Social History of American Medicine*, ed. Morris J. Vogel and Charles E. Rosenberg (Philadelphia: University of Pennsylvania Press, 1979), esp. pp. 211–12.

12.   Sophia F. Palmer, "Women in the War," SS 1899, p. 70, quoting September 1898 statement by McGee; McGee to [Sophia] Palmer, Dec. 12, 1900, Army Nurse Corps Historical Files, Record Group 112, National Archives, Washington, D.C. (collection hereafter cited as ANC Files, Archives.)

13.   Anita Newcomb McGee to Amy Wingreen, June 9, 1898, Amy Wingreen Papers, Newberry Library, Chicago; [McGee], Memo [Fall 1898?], ANC Files, Archives; McGee, "Standard for Army Nurses," *TN* 22

(April 1899): 172 explained McGee's preference for graduate nurses. The rationale for choosing nurses from all geographical areas is presented in McGee, "Co-Relation of Nurses' Organizations," *TN* 23 (November 1899): 296; Kinney, "Dr. McGee," *TN* 26 (March 1901): 131; McGee to Senator William Allison, March 3, 1899, ANC Files, Archives; cf. Gerald F. Linderman, *The Mirror of War: American Society and the Spanish-American War* (Ann Arbor: University of Michigan Press, 1974), p. 70 (hereafter cited as Linderman, *Mirror*). On the nurses employed, see "The Public Service: Report of the Surgeon General of the Army," *Journal of the American Medical Association* (hereafter cited as *JAMA*) 33 (Nov. 25, 1899): 1377; Dock, *Red Cross*, p. 43.

14. McGee to [Sophia] Palmer, May 11, 1899; McGee to Miss Peters, June 19, 1900, both in ANC Files, Archives. For nurses' comments on conditions in army hospitals, see Helen W. Bissell, "A Woman's View of Chickamauga," June 21, 1899, Army Nursing Boxes, Nightingale Room, Welch Medical Library, Johns Hopkins University, Baltimore (hereafter cited as Army Nursing, Welch); Mrs. H. C. Lounsbery, "Some Reminiscences of Sternberg Hospital," *AJN* 3 (October 1902): 1–5; L. W. Quintard, "The Field Hospital at Camp Wikoff," *SS* 1899, pp. 81–88. P. M. Ashburn, *A History of the Medical Department of the United States Army*, with an introduction by Surgeon General Merritte W. Ireland (Boston: Houghton Mifflin Co., 1929), p. 208 n. 1, quotes a letter revealing an army physician's initial distrust of nurses and his growing respect for them.

15. Quotation from Elisabeth Mills Reid, Katherine W. Ambrose Shrady, "Auxiliary No. 3," in *Relief Committee Reports*, p. 41. For signs of war enthusiasm, see Linderman, *Mirror*, pp. 63–64, 73–74, and *Relief Committee Reports*, pp. v–vi, 1–3.

16.   "Mrs. Cowdin's Death," *New York Times*, Oct. 20, 1906, p. 9; Dock, *Red Cross*, p. 48; NAW, s.v. "Reid, Elisabeth Mills," by Raymond S. Milowski; *Dictionary of American Biography*, s.v. "Mills, Darius Ogden," by Alexander D. Noyes; s.v. "Reid, Whitelaw," by Allan Nevins; Dorothy Giles, *A Candle in Her Hand: A Story of the Nursing Schools of Bellevue Hospital* (New York: G. P. Putnam's Sons, 1949), p. 228. Reid was off the Bellevue board between 1889 and 1893. The quotation on Cowles's dislike of publicity is from Isabel McIsaac to Adelaide Nutting, Dec. 9, [1901], Army Nursing, Welch. On Cowles, see "Mrs. W. S. Cowles Dies At Age of 76," *New York Times*, Aug. 26, 1931, p. 19; Lillian Rixey, *Bamie: Theodore Roosevelt's Remarkable Sister* (New York: David McKay Co., 1963), esp. p. 19.

17. Reid, Shrady, "Auxiliary No. 3," in *Relief Committee Reports*, pp. 41–43; including the quoted description of President William McKinley's help, p. 43; cf. "Hospital Notes," *TN* 21 (August 1898): 116. The quotation about having McGee certify the Auxiliary's nurses is from "Red Cross Nurses," *TN* 21 (September 1898): 164; Reid, Shrady, "Auxiliary No. 3," in *Relief Committee Reports*, pp. 48–49, 52–53.

18. See Reid, Shrady, "Auxiliary No. 3," in *Relief Committee Reports*, p. 41, for the quotations on graduates of standing and superintendents' assistance; see pp. 46, 47, 48, 50, 51, on the careful provision of superintendents for contingents of nurses. Dock, *Red Cross*, p. 50, mentions the committee of superintendents. Although belated, her account was based on interviews and correspondence with participants, as well as documents. Robb, "Lessons," p. 153, cf. p. 154.

19. The quotation is from Robb, "Lessons," p. 156. On the meeting, see "Lessons," pp. 156–57; Anna C. Maxwell, "The Field Hospital at Chickamauga Park," SS 1899, pp. 76–77; Executive Committee Meeting of NAA, Dec. 28, 1898, Board of Directors Minutes, American Nurses' Association Records, Nursing History Archive, Mugar Memorial Library, Boston University, Boston (collection hereafter cited as ANA, BU.) Three documents give the slightly changing membership of the committee as of 1899, 1900, and 1901. "Committee to Secure by Act of Congress the Employment of Graduate Women Nurses in the Hospital Service of the United States Army," Leaflet [1899], "Committee to Secure . . . ," Leaflet [1900], both in ANC Files, Archives; "Final Report of the Committee to Secure . . . ," Minutes, Feb. 8, 1901, Army Nursing, Welch. Most members of the committee are identified in the leaflets cited, *Relief Committee Reports*, p. 39, or Dock, *Red Cross*, pp. 67–68. See also NAW, s.v. "Richards, Linda," by Stella Goostray, and *Directory of the National Society of the Daughters of the American Revolution, Compiled by Order of the Tenth Continental Congress* (Washington, D.C.: n.p., 1901), p. 596 (on Mrs. W. N. Armstrong).

20. The lay committee members' roles are evident in "Nurses for Regular Army: House Committee Agrees on Bill for Permanent Corps," *Washington Post*, Feb. 4, 1899, p. 4; "Women as Army Nurses," *New York Tribune*, Feb. 4, 1899, p. 7; Maxwell, "Hospital at Chickamauga," SS 1899, p. 77. "A Bill. To provide for the employment of women nurses in military hospitals of the Army" was endorsed in McGee's hand, "Submitted to S. G. Nov. 15–99, in person by Mrs. Cowdin and Mrs. Cutting," ANC Files, Archives. (Cutting was an Auxiliary No. 3 veteran on the Bill Committee.) McGee to Mrs. Winthrop Cowdin, March 6, 1899, and McGee to Mrs. Rose, Nov. 20, 1899, both in ANC Files, Archives, refer to visits to legislators and officials, one by non-nurse members of the Bill Committee, the other by two nurses and Cowdin. "Final Report," Feb. 8, 1901, Army Nursing, Welch, suggests that most contacts with legislators were handled by the laywomen. Nurses' efforts to win support for the bill are revealed in "Pennsylvania," *JAMA* 34 (March 10, 1900): 632; "Pennsylvania," *JAMA* 34 (March 17, 1900): 698; Linda Richards to Adelaide Nutting, n.d., Feb. 16, 1900, Feb. 19, 1900, March 2, 1900, all in Army Nursing, Welch; McGee to Anna M. Peters, May 3, 1900, ANC Files, Archives; "Association News," *JAMA* 32 (June 10, 1899): 1336, 1338. "Not a Mistake," Editorial, TN 23 (December 1899): 405, claimed that Robb, wife of a physician, arranged for pre-

sentation of the bill to the American Medical Association. Maxwell, "Hospital at Chickamauga," *SS* 1899, p. 77. However, two other nurse members of the Bill Committee indicated that both nurses and laywomen participated in drafting the bill: Robb, "Lessons," p. 157, and "The Army Nursing Bill," *Seventh Annual Report of the Alumnae Association of the Johns Hopkins Hospital Training School for Nurses, 1898–1899*, p. 4, in Mary Adelaide Nutting Papers, Nightingale Room, Welch Medical Library, Johns Hopkins University, Baltimore.

21.   Executive Committee Meeting of NAA, Dec. 28, 1898, ANA, BU; "An Act to Provide for the Employment of Women Nurses in Military Hospitals of the Army," endorsed S. 5353, H.R. 11770, enclosed with Judith E. Foster [counsel to the Bill Committee], to McGee, Jan. 24, 1899, ANC Files, Archives; U.S. Congress, House, Mr. Griffin introducing H.R. 11770, 55th Cong., 3rd sess., Jan. 24, 1899; and U.S. Congress, Senate, Mr. Burrows introducing S. 5353, 55th Cong., 3rd sess., Jan. 25, 1899, both in *Congressional Record* 32:1013, 1016. On salaries, see "Surgeon General Sternberg's Report on the Bill for the Employment of Female Army Nurses," *TN* 22 (March 1899): 125; Helen E. Marshall, *Mary Adelaide Nutting: Pioneer of Modern Nursing* (Baltimore: Johns Hopkins University Press, 1972), p. 67 (hereafter cited as Marshall, *Pioneer*). On NAA membership, see Flanagan, *Voice*, pp. 44–47.

22.   The quotations describing nurses are from Maxwell, "Hospital at Chickamauga," *SS* 1899, p. 76; Robb, "Lessons," p. 159, quoting a supporter or member of the Bill Committee, cf. Quintard, "Hospital at Wikoff," *SS* 1899, p. 87. The quotation about having a nurse as superintendent is from "Women as Army Nurses," *New York Tribune*, Feb. 4, 1899, p. 7. The proposed all-woman commission is outlined in "Association News," *JAMA* 32 (June 10, 1899): 1336.

23.   On congressional disgust with the Medical Department, see John M. Gibson, *Soldier in White: The Life of General George Miller Sternberg* (Durham, N.C.: Duke University Press, 1958), pp. 197–208; and U.S. Congress, House, Discussion and vote on H.R. 11770, 55th Cong., 3rd sess., Feb. 6, 1899, *Congressional Record* 32:1513–18. For examples of criticisms of the bill by Surgeon General Sternberg and McGee, see "Trained Female Nurses for the Army," *JAMA* 32 (Feb. 11, 1899): 329; "Surgeon General Sternberg's Report," *TN* 22 (March 1899): 123–25; "The Contract Nurse Bill," *JAMA* 32 (Feb. 18, 1899): 389. "Committee to Secure . . . ," Leaflet [1900], ANC Files, Archives contains the text of H.R. 6879, S. 2699. U.S. Congress, House, Mr. Hull introducing H.R. 6879, 56th Cong., 1st sess., Jan. 19, 1900; U.S. Congress, Senate, Mr. Hawley introducing S. 2699, 56th Cong., 1st sess., Jan. 25, 1900, both in *Congressional Record* 33; 1010, 1155. The quotation is from Minutes, General Committee to Secure . . . , May 26, 1900, Army Nursing, Welch. [Anita Newcomb McGee], Draft of Provi-

sion for Army Nurse Corps, Nov. 12, 1900, ANC Files, Archives; McGee, "Legislation for Army Nurses," *TN* 26 (April 1901): 208; U.S. Congress, Senate, Discussion and vote on Section 19, S. 4300, 56th Cong., 2nd sess., Jan. 4, 1901, *Congressional Record* 34:549.

24. McGee's support of equal opportunity for graduates of nonelite training schools appears in McGee, "Standard," *TN* 22 (April 1899): 173–74 and in [McGee], "Notes Regarding H.R. 6879," enclosed with McGee to Senator Redfield Proctor, March 5, 1900, ANC Files, Archives, which was published with only slight alterations as a *Philadelphia Medical Journal* editorial, reprinted in "Some Editorial Comments on the Army Nursing Bill," *TN* 24 (May 1900): 366–68. For rank-and-file nurse agreement with McGee's position on this issue, see Katherine A. Sherry to editor, *TN* 22 (June 1899): 318; Lillian M. Kratz to editor, *TN* 25 (September 1900): 204–5; Susan B. Read to editor, *TN* 23 (December 1899): 403. A letter to individual members of House and Senate Military Affairs Committees, Feb. 14, 1900, on *Trained Nurse* stationery, ANC Files, Archives, claimed that after publication of an antibill letter in December the magazine received two hundred letters from nurses opposing army nursing legislation. DAR President General Mrs. Daniel Manning is quoted in "Women as Army Nurses," *New York Tribune*, Feb. 4, 1899, p. 7. The quotation about serving Illinois troops is from Gertrude G. Wellington to McGee, May 28, 1898, in McGee, "Co-Relation of Nurses' Organizations," *TN* 23 (November 1899): 295.

25. "Final Report of the Committee . . . ," Feb. 8, 1901, Army Nursing, Welch; Dock, *Red Cross*, pp. 87–97; Mabel T. Boardman, *Under the Red Cross Flag at Home and Abroad*, with a foreword by Woodrow Wilson, 2nd ed. (Philadelphia: J. B. Lippincott Co., 1917), pp. 46–64, 97–98, description of Sanitary Commission in chapter title, p. 46; Foster Rhea Dulles, *The American Red Cross: A History* (New York: Harper & Bros., 1950), pp. 64–71; "Nursing News and Announcements," *AJN* 10 (February 1910): 350.

26. M. Louise Fitzpatrick, *The National Organization for Public Health Nursing, 1912–1952: Development of a Practice Field* (New York: National League for Nursing, 1975), pp. 17, 24–25 (hereafter cited as Fitzpatrick, *NOPHN*). On the registration movement, see, for example, James H. Rodabaugh and Mary Jane Rodabaugh, *Nursing in Ohio: A History* (Columbus: Ohio State Nurses' Association, 1951), pp. 93–103; Carla M. Schissel, "The State Nurses' Association in a Georgia Context, 1907–1946" (Ph.D. dissertation, Emory University, 1979), pp. 7–48. Organized nurses' imitation of physicians and cultivation of ties with them did not mean relations were always harmonious; in some states physicians and their groups were important foes of registration. October 1916 statement by Wilson, quoted in Martin, *Digest*, pp. 41–42. On the CND system as in part the creation of self-conscious professionals eager to organize American society,

see Robert D. Cuff, *The War Industries Board: Business-Government Relations During World War I* (Baltimore: Johns Hopkins University Press, 1973), pp. 13–42.

27. The quotations are from Minutes, Advisory Council and Executive Committee, NOPHN, May 4, 1917, Lillian D. Wald Papers, New York Public Library (hereafter cited as Wald Papers, NYPL). Minutes, Advisory Council and Executive Committee, NOPHN, June 4, 1917; Mary Beard to Directors and Advisory Council, NOPHN, [late July 1917]; Beard to Dr. George Vincent, [December 1917?], all in Wald Papers, NYPL; Portia B. Kernodle, *The Red Cross Nurse in Action, 1882–1948* (New York: Harper & Bros., 1949), pp. 126–27 (hereafter cited as Kernodle, *Red Cross Nurse*).

28. "The Reminiscences of Isabel Maitland Stewart," Oral History Research Office, Columbia University, 1961, pp. 178–79 (hereafter cited as Stewart, "Reminiscences"); Marshall, *Pioneer*, pp. 223–24, 226–27. For the committee's actions, see "The National Crisis and the College-Trained Woman," *Modern Hospital* (hereafter cited as *MH*) 9 (July 1917): 31–32; "A Survey of Nursing Resources," *MH* 9 (August 1917): 127; "Purpose, Program and Personnel of Committee on Nursing, General Medical Board," [Summer 1917], ANC Files, Archives. On relations between the Committee on Nursing and the CND, see Martin, *Digest*, pp. 236, 240, 455–56, 462; "National Defense Committee Supports Nursing Standards," Editorial, *AJN* 18 (December 1917): 185–86; Franklin Martin and F. F. Simpson to training-school superintendents, [1917], ANC Files, Archives.

29. Nancy Tomes, "A Collision of Nursing's Two Worlds: Volunteer and Professional Nursing in World War I" (Paper presented at the Conference on Women in the Health Professions, Boston College, Nov. 15, 1980), offers a full and illuminating account of this episode. For objections to aids, see Stewart, "Reminiscences," p. 175; Clara D. Noyes statement, Minutes of 18th Annual Convention, ANA, June 21, 1915, ANA, BU; Elizabeth Burgess, "The Readjustment of the Curriculum to Meet War Needs and Its Effects upon the Hospitals," National League of Nursing Education, *Proceedings of the Twenty-Fourth Annual Convention* [1918] (Baltimore: Williams & Wilkins Co., 1919), pp. 146–47 (proceedings hereafter identified by *NLNE* and the year of the convention). On training of aids, see "The Red Cross Home Nursing Courses," *MH* 9 (August 1917): 131; Kernodle, *Red Cross Nurse*, pp. 111–12, 124, 135–36. On the situation in early 1918, see David M. Kennedy, *Over Here: The First World War and American Society* (New York: Oxford University Press, 1980), pp. 169–70. J. W. McConaughy to Secretary of War, "Confidential Memo," Jan. 26, 1918; [McConaughy], "Memorandum for Secretary Baker. Army Nurse Corps" [January or February 1918]; Baker to Surgeon General Gorgas, "Confidential," Feb. 7, 1918, all in ANC Files, Archives; Annie W. Goodrich, "The Plan for the Army School of Nursing," *NLNE* 1918, p. 172; Kernodle, *Red Cross Nurse*, pp. 135–36. Hospital spokesmen's clamor for

aids reached a peak in the spring of 1918. See, for example, Martin, *Digest*, pp. 382, describing a March 10, 1918, GMB meeting; "Call for Women as Nurses' Aids," *New York Times*, April 17, 1918, p. 12; "Many City Nurses Taken by the War," *New York Times*, May 15, 1918, p. 24; "The Nursing Profession and the National Crisis," Editorial, *MH* 10 (April 1918): 275–76.

30. The quoted phrases are from Goodrich, "Army School," *NLNE* 1918, p. 172; Goodrich, "The Contribution of the Army School of Nursing," *NLNE* 1919, pp. 152–53, quoting her 1918 report recommending establishment of the Army School. Goodrich, in discussion, *NLNE* 1918, p. 187; Nutting, *Economic Basis*, pp. 3–39; Goodrich, *Significance*, pp. 27–61.

31. Jane A. Delano, "Red Cross Aid Versus the Short-Term Course," *NLNE* 1918, pp. 159–71; vote on the school, *NLNE* 1918, 190–92. Two (physician) hospital administrators, both members of Nutting's CND Committee, also addressed the convention on the issue. S. S. Goldwater, "The Nursing Crisis: Efforts to Satisfy the Nursing Requirements of the War," *NLNE* 1918, pp. 132–39, advocated training and military use of aids; Winford H. Smith, "How Nurses Are Meeting the Present Needs," *AJN* 18 (August 1918): 979–86, supported the Army School. "Shall We Have An Army School of Nursing?" Editorial, *AJN* 18 (June 1918): 764; Minutes, Committee on Nursing, General Medical Board, May 27, 1918, ANC Files, Archives; Martin, *Digest*, p. 430; David Loth, *A Long Way Forward: The Biography of Congresswoman Frances P. Bolton* (New York: Longmans, Green & Co., 1957), pp. 104–8 (hereafter cited as Loth, *Bolton*); Kernodle, *Red Cross Nurse*, pp. 138–39.

32. Isabel McIsaac to Adelaide Nutting, Nov. 13, [1901], Army Nursing, Welch, in reference to efforts to improve the standing of nurses in the newly established ANC. Loth, *Bolton*, pp. 61, 64–66, 70–72, 82; Fitzpatrick, *NOPHN*, p. 61; Frances Payne Bolton, "Voluntary Aid in Nursing—What It Is and What It Is Not," *Public Health Nurse Quarterly* 10 (April 1918): 129–32, quotation p. 129.

33. Bolton, in discussion, *NLNE* 1918, p. 182.

34. Dora E. Thompson, "How the Army Nursing Service Met the Demands of the War," *NLNE* 1919, pp. 116–17, reported that when the United States declared war there were 233 ANC members and 170 reserve nurses on duty; at the armistice there were 21,498 on duty. The reference to serfdom is in Sarah [*sic*] E. Parsons, "Impressions and Conclusions Based on Experience Abroad by Overseas Nurses," *NLNE* 1919, p. 168; for the standard complaints, see "Discussion on Rank," *AJN* 19 (August 1919): 851–53. Philip A. Kalisch, "How Army Nurses Became Officers," *Nursing Research* (hereafter cited as *NR*) 25 (May–June 1976): 164–77, offers a detailed and valuable account of the rank campaign with emphasis on Nutting's role but no attention to the suffragist contribution. Resolution of May 1917 ANA convention, quoted in Dock, *Red Cross*, pp. 1064–65.

35. "Raise War Nurses' Rank," *Woman Citizen* 1, n.s. (July 14,

1917): 121, refers to a June resolution by the College Equal Suffrage League; Helen Hoy Greeley, "The Lewis-Baker [Raker] Bill," *WJM* 29 (May 1919): 83; Dock, *Red Cross*, p. 1065; *NAW*, s.v. "Havemeyer, Louisine Waldron Elder," by Neil Harris. While the traditions of the ANC were being established McGee wanted the superintendent given the officer's rank that she, being a physician, enjoyed during her stint in the Medical Department. She chided the Bill Committee for ignoring rank and apparently discussed the question of the proper rank for ordinary ANC members with her successor. McGee to [Sophia] Palmer, May 11, 1899, Dec. 12, 1900; Dita Kinney to [McGee], Dec. 6, 1907, all in ANC Files, Archives; Anita Newcomb McGee, "Army Nurse Corps," in *A Reference Handbook of the Medical Sciences*, new ed., rev., ed. Albert H. Buck, 9 vols. (New York: W. Wood & Co., 1900–1908); 1:517; Georgia Nevins to Isabel [Robb?], June 7, 1899, Army Nursing, Welch, reporting a conversation with McGee.

For the wartime activities of suffrage militants, see Inez Haynes Irwin, *The Story of the Woman's Party* (New York: Harcourt, Brace & Co., 1921), pp. 196–220. Unlike Blatch, Havemeyer did picket and go to jail; see ibid., pp. 402–7. Blatch's autobiography does not mention the rank campaign but does justify her decision to substitute war work for suffrage agitation, Harriot Stanton Blatch and Alma Lutz, *Challenging Years: The Memoirs of Harriot Stanton Blatch* (New York: G. P. Putnam's Sons, 1940), pp. 283–85; on her interest in working women, see pp. 92–94, 98, on association with Greeley, pp. 94, 108, 115. Dock, *Red Cross*, pp. 1065–66. Kalisch, "Officers," *NR* 25 (May–June 1976): 164–65, citing Nutting to Martin, Oct. 26, 1917, and a recommendation from Nutting to Secretary of War Baker in January 1917. I assume that this is a misprint for 1918, since the United States was not at war in January 1917.

36. "Seek Rank for Women Doctors in the War Zone," Editorial, *WMJ* 28 (March 1918): 63, refers to a resolution by a patriotic women's group favoring rank for nurses as well as women physicians; Minutes, Board of Directors, ANA, NLNE, and NOPHN, May 6, 1918, microfilm reel 2, National League for Nursing, New York, refers to support for rank by the "Intercollegiate Alumnae." Harriot Stanton Blatch to editor, *New York Times*, March 9, 1918, p. 14; William Montague Geer to editor, *New York Times*, March 11, 1918, p. 10; George Gordon Battle to editor, *New York Times*, March 26, 1918, p. 10; "Rank and Title Their Due," Editorial, *New York Times*, March 12, 1918, p. 12; Martin, *Digest*, pp. 387–88, and see p. 462.

37. "Nurses Ask Military Rank," *Washington Post*, April 16, 1918, p. 4; "Nurses Ask Military Rank," *Washington Post*, April 17, 1918, p. 3; Dock, *Red Cross*, pp. 1066–76. "Ask Army Rank for Nurses," *New York Times*, April 26, 1918, p. 13, reported that a newspaperwoman and the wives of a former mayor of New York and newspaperman William Randolph Hearst led a group testifying in favor of rank. Their connection with other participants in the campaign is unclear, but it is notable that, like the suf-

fragists, they were not wealthy philanthropists of the type of Elisabeth Reid or Frances Bolton. "Nurses above Sergeants," *New York Times*, Aug. 11, 1918, sec. 1, p. 3. "Proceedings of the Twenty-First Annual Convention of the American Nurses' Association," *AJN* 18 (July 1918): 962–63; May 1918 resolution, National League of Nursing Education records, microfilm reel 2, National League for Nursing, New York.

38.   On Greeley's role and activities, see Minutes, Board of Directors, NOPHN, May 11, 1918, Wald Papers, NYPL, which contains the phrase "work with Mrs. Greeley"; Minutes, Committee on Nursing, General Medical Board, May 27, 1918, ANC Files, Archives. Kalisch, "Officers," NR 25 (May–June 1976): 172, quotes Greeley's offer to defer pay, Greeley to Nutting, Jan. 2, 1919. Greeley, "Rank for Nurses," *AJN* 19 (August 1919): 846–47, 849; Greeley, "Rank for Nurses," *NLNE* 1918, pp. 298–303; Martin, *Digest*, p. 416. Palmer's statement is in Kalisch, "Officers," NR 25 (May–June 1976): 172, quoting Palmer to Nutting, April 15, 1919. [Julia Stimson], "History of the American Army Nurse Corps and Its Work During the World War," [1920], ANC Files, Archives; Greeley to "Fellow-Worker for Rank," Aug. 18, 1920, Lillian D. Wald Papers, Columbia University, New York.

39.   Delano is quoted in U.S. Congress, House, material inserted by Mr. Raker, 66th Cong., 2nd sess., March 9, 1920, *Congressional Record* 59: 4097. For similar arguments, see letters to editor from Martha M. Russell, R. Inde Allbaugh, Annie W. Goodrich, A. M. Hilliard, M. A. Nutting, and M. M. Riddle, *AJN* 19 (July 1919): 796–800; Elizabeth Folckemer, "Efficiency in the Army Nurse Corps," *Public Health Nurse* 11 (November 1919): 920–23. In the 1920s and 1930s nurse leaders did develop an interest in the scientific-management approach to efficiency, see Susan Reverby, "The Search for the Hospital Yardstick: Nursing and the Rationalization of Hospital Work," in *Health Care in America: Essays in Social History*, ed. Susan Reverby and David Rosner (Philadelphia: Temple University Press, 1979), pp. 206–25.

40.   "Military Rank for Army Nurses," *Survey* 40 (Sept. 21, 1918): 698; Kalisch, "Officers," NR 25 (May–June 1976): 171–72, quoting Greeley to Nutting, Jan. 2, 1919.

41.   Clara D. Noyes to editor, *AJN* 19 (April 1919): 553–55, quotation p. 554.

42.   U.S. Congress, House, Mr. Raker speaking in favor of provision for relative rank included in H.R. 12775, 66th Cong., 2nd sess., March 9, 1920, *Congressional Record* 59:4093; "Some Quotations from the Hearings Before the Sub-Committee of the Committee on Military Affairs, United States Senate," *AJN* 20 (October 1919): 34–38; Greeley to "Fellow-Worker for Rank," Aug. 18, 1920, Wald Papers, Columbia; Kalisch, "Officers," NR 25 (May–June 1976): 171.

43.   "Some Quotations from Hearings," *AJN* 20 (October 1919): 30–34; Dock, *Red Cross*, pp. 1069, 1072–73.

3

Professionalizing Strategies as Time- and Culture-Bound: American and British Nursing, Circa 1893

Celia Davies

During the past summer I have had the opportunity of a conversation with a lady of great practical experience in nursing, and one of the most noted and influential living advocates of the utility of training schools for the education of nurses. I allude, as you will infer, to FLORENCE NIGHTINGALE.

These were the words of Dr. Joseph Toner, president of the Washington Training School for Nurses, in his address at the school's fourth convocation in 1881. He described, in enthusiastic detail, how he had delivered to Florence Nightingale's home a set of photographs of the successful graduates of the school and a plate, cup, and saucer especially decorated for an exhibition in aid of the school. He read, in full, Nightingale's note of thanks and her invitation to a meeting. Listeners learned that the presents had been set out on a small writing table at the time of the visit; they heard a full description of Nightingale herself (including even an estimate of her weight), as well as a report of her views on schools and on the matter of nurses for the poor. The *Washington Evening Star* decided that this address was of such interest that it merited a verbatim report. The address took four columns of print, three of which were devoted entirely to Nightingale. The doctor's tone was admiring and respectful. Florence Nightingale was a leading figure and a noble example to others.[1]

47

The visit of this American medical man was not an isolated incident. Florence Nightingale had many American callers. Dr. Emily Blackwell, who, with her sister Elizabeth, had founded the New York Infirmary for Women and Children in 1854, returned from a visit to Nightingale with new ideas for reforms in 1861. Dr. W. Gill Wylie, of the Bellevue Hospital, owing to a mishap, failed in his intention to meet Nightingale before the setting up of the nurse training school there, but a close correspondence with her was quickly initiated and maintained. Francis King, president of the Board of Trustees of the new Johns Hopkins Hospital, was more successful when he traveled to England in 1875 to see both Nightingale and the school she had influenced so much. Later, American nurse leaders also visited. Isabel Hampton, who became superintendent of the renowned Johns Hopkins School of Nursing in 1889 and was to play a leading part in the formation of American nursing associations, paid her respects in 1894, on the eve of her marriage to Dr. Hunter Robb. Adelaide Nutting, who was in the first class at Hopkins and who was later to be the first nurse to hold a full professorship, was a caller at the famous house in South Street in 1902. Furthermore, though Florence Nightingale herself was confined to her sickroom from the 1860s onward, nurses from the Nightingale school and from other British schools traveled to the United States, and some took up posts there. At the turn of the century, then, Nightingale's ideas and her personal stature stimulated a considerable transatlantic exchange of visitors.[2]

Despite this to and fro, however, American nursing was no carbon copy of the Nightingale system. Not only did American training schools quickly diverge from patterns established by their British counterparts, but American nurse leaders also developed interesting and distinctive forms of professional organization. Indeed, it is for the insights one can gain into the features of organized nursing as it developed in the United States that a cross-cultural, comparative perspective is most helpful.

Several matters of methods are essential to the comparisons I shall draw. In particular, it is important to note that while I shall use the concepts of *professional ideology* and *professionalizing strategy*, I shall not employ the concept of *professionalization*. This requires brief explanation.

In their studies of the professions and of the process of professionalization, scholars have been neither always consistent nor always clear. To some, professionalization has meant a sequence of specific events (the adoption of a title, the setting up of a school, and so on). Laudable at the least for its clarity, this approach to the question of professionalization has been criticized and rejected by an increasing number of sociologists and historians because it is too tied to time and place to serve as a basis for generalizing about occupations. For this, and for other reasons, an insistence that professions and the process of professionalization are "about power" has become more fashionable. Yet this approach also raises almost as many questions as it answers. Can professionalization take different specific forms, and, if so, how do we recognize it when it occurs? Are there other ways in which occupations develop, and, if so, what are they? Under what circumstances does each occur? It may be altogether too much of a simplification to insist that all occupational activity is "about power."[3]

As a general concept, then, "professionalization" may confuse more than it clarifies, although the stubborn point remains that all kinds of ideas about professions abound in the worlds we study, and we ignore them at our peril. This is where the concepts of professional ideology and of professionalizing strategy enter. They are useful in dealing precisely with the ideas that organize the aspirations and activities of the actors involved, and the behaviors that follow.

Let me specify these terms a little more formally. I would define *professional ideology* as referring to the interpretative and explanatory statements offered by leaders of an occupational group concerning their activities (individual and collective) qua members. Relevant statements relate to (*a*) the nature and worth of the activities in which they jointly engage and (*b*) the matrix of social relations in which their activities are to be located. Statements may also provide a logic to link (*a*) and (*b*). *Professionalizing strategy*, by contrast, refers to the collective actions of leaders of an occupational group designed by them to institutionalize activities and relations pertaining to them as a group. The devices they propose may be directly political—aiming at participation, influence, regulation, and so forth, or they may be indirectly so, being ways of defining and associating members. My claim is that ideology links to strategy, helping to define a program of action and rendering action both comprehensible and achievable.[4]

One final point is in order before leaving these definitions. It will be observed both in respect to ideology and in respect to strategy that a leadership is specifically mentioned. The professional ideology is a leader ideology, the strategy a leader strategy, or rather, it is the "official" view as propounded by leaders. Why is it important to qualify in this way and what are the implications of doing so? Perhaps more than many other occupational groups, nursing embraces a variety of different positions as far as market chances, status, and power are concerned. Leaders may try to level this or they may not. Either way their expressed ideologies for the group are not likely to be identical to those of the rank and file, nor are their strategies for the group likely always to be received with enthusiasm. Indeed the leaders' dilemma in nursing (and perhaps in other stratified occupational groups) lies precisely in this: how simultaneously to enhance the position of the group and the position of themselves as an elite within the group. That the occupational group as a social formation persists suggests that this somehow has been achieved. That aside, references to an "official" ideology or to "official" strategy are not to be equated with the beliefs or sanctioned behaviors of all members of the occupational group.

NURSING STRATEGY EXPOUNDED

The year 1893 marks the point at which American nurses first came together to design organizations and activities that, they hoped, would alter their collective fate. The occasion was the International Congress of Charities, Corrections and Philanthropy in Chicago, Illinois. Two organizational devices emerged from the meetings of the section on Hospitals, Dispensaries, and Nursing. One, worked out in detail immediately, was the Society of Superintendents of Training Schools for Nurses, later to be extended and renamed the National League of Nursing Education. The other was the Nurses Associated Alumnae, a body that was set up three years later and was to develop into the American Nurses' Association.[5]

The events of 1893 were clearly part of a plan, deliberately conceived by a group of women who were to become important leaders of American nursing. Among these were Isabel Hampton Robb and Adelaide Nutting, both of whom, as we have noted, had been at Johns Hopkins, and Lavinia Dock, a graduate of Bellevue who had begun at Johns Hopkins as assistant to Hampton in 1890. Various sources suggest that they had met to plan the meeting itself, and there is little doubt that their thinking and discussion had been developing throughout the period of Hampton's tenure as superintendent of nurses at Johns Hopkins Hospital and even before. So well rehearsed were the plans by the time of the meeting that Hampton was able to sum up from the chair, outlining a clear plan of campaign. She put it as follows:

> Superintendents being the heads of schools have a great deal of influence, not only among their pupils, but graduate nurses, and until we can get Superintendents united regarding the fundamental

principles of the work, we cannot expect the nurses to work and to unite and to be as successful as they must be later when we hold ideas in common. The next thing we can take steps towards accomplishing is to organize a Superintendents' Society and also alumnae associations in connection with every good school in the country. The alumnae associations should be as nearly alike as possible. . . . I do not think superintendents should take too active a part. . . . Until these alumnae associations are in good working order it will be impossible to organize a national association because in that we must have schools and hospitals and nurses represented.[6]

Let us look at this plan in a little more detail and as a professionalizing strategy. The major solution being put forward emphasized voluntaristic change. It counseled self-help and it assumed that superintendents, with the support of like-minded colleagues, would grasp the nettle of change. Superintendents, speakers urged, should come out of their isolation. They should visit other schools; together they should discuss good practice. The position emerged that the formation of a society could make known the best in current practice; it could be a forum for the expression of new ideas; and it could provide support for innovators. With its encouragement, poor schools could become good, and good schools better. The plan assumed enthusiasm, hard work, and personal involvement. On its own, however, this was not enough. Good schools should have their own associations of alumnae, organized not by superintendents but by trained nurses themselves. Out of these associations, in a way as yet unspecified, a national membership organization would grow.

Further addresses at the congress developed the idea of organizing alumnae. Isobel McIsaac, the assistant superintendent at Illinois Training School, Chicago, explained that a key rationale for alumnae associations was to be found in the mutual help they afforded to graduate nurses, and the possibility of further educational activities. Another speaker, Edith Draper, superintendent of the Illinois School, mused on what a national organization could do by way of extending and consolidating the alumnae work that nurses were already finding valuable. Financial and educational benefits were stressed, as was the value of unifying nursing and providing contacts for the graduate nurse, who, ten years out of school, might feel out of touch with developments. The speaker was careful to stress the uplifting possibilities of such an association and to dispel any notion that collective action could be seen in any way as degrading. This was echoed by Irene Sutcliffe from New York

Hospital, who wondered whether a well-regulated association of nurses might not do much toward correcting the danger of losing ideals.[7]

It was the Superintendents' Society, however, that was the real rallying point of the meetings. Other organizational plans were discussed, such as the formation of alumnae associations, but they were dealt with more tentatively. Why was the Superintendents' Society considered so important? We will be in a better position to account for this when we have looked more closely at the nurses' interpretations of the position of their profession at this time and of the way in which they had arrived at this point.

A considerable amount of time at the congress was taken up by the various speakers' efforts to make sense of the then current situation in nursing. The most prominent feature for comment was the expansion and proliferation of training schools. And no wonder. So rapidly had the schools opened their doors that the "trained nurse" had become a familiar figure within the space of less than twenty years. Seven years later she was even recognized in the *U.S. Census*, when a category of "trained nurse" was added to the occupational classifications.[8]

Of course, the training schools had not been established as a result of activity by nurses. Various parties had been involved and motives for setting them up were a complex mixture of philanthropic ideals, personal interests, and, increasingly as far as the hospitals were concerned, sheer economic sense. What is striking about the accounts given in 1893, therefore, especially in the light of recent writings on nurse training, with their strong emphasis on economic factors and the economic exploitation of nurses, is that the self-interest of training-school founders as a factor in the setting up of schools was *not* emphasized by the nurses. Instead the need for initiatives from nurses themselves was stressed. And the gross differences of standards that were apparent to all were not attributed to the recalcitrance of school managements or to a conflict of material interests. The need for initiative by nurses was stressed. "Our founders achieved well and nobly," Isabel Hampton insisted. "But surely it was not intended that we should work forever on the old lines?"[9]

How, then, were nurses to begin to work on new lines? How were they to exercise increasing responsibility for their field of work? No one at the congress was arguing for unity of ideas or for the imposition of a standard on lagging schools. Taking a benign look at the past, and emphasizing, as so many occupational histories and historians do, positive achievements and individual contributions, Isabel Hampton said: "Each school is a law unto itself. Nothing in the way of unity of ideas or of general principles to govern all exists, and no effort towards establishing and maintaining a general standard for all has ever been attempted." Progress through encouragement rather than sanctions was a keynote of much that was urged at the conference.[10]

The emphasis on voluntary reforms rather than coercion was evident, not only in the nurses' somewhat uncritical view of their past, but also in the comparisons they drew with nursing in Britain. The paper presented by Louise Darche, superintendent of the New York City Training School, is particularly important here. She argued, in effect, that the pattern of development of nursing in Britain was not the same as in the United States and that the differences were such as to necessitate a different strategy.

Darche drew attention to the point that at St. Thomas's Hospital in London, a nurse trained for one year and was pledged to remain in the service of the training committee for a further three years. The nurse was never given a certificate and never apparently gained full independence. This was puzzling to an American, and Darche mused: ". . . it would seem that the nurse is never graduated in the sense of being placed on her own responsibility, but must always remain under the supervising control and authority of the training committee." Such a system, she went on to argue, was unthinkable in the United States, "where the idea of pledging oneself to a corporation or society for a period of four years, not to say indefinitely, would have been regarded as impossible." The point was this: the viability of the arrangement had allowed Nightingale to send out teams of nurses to make improvements in other hospitals. It was justifiable and it had had results, but it was not something that could be accomplished in the same way in America. The strong implication was that some other arrangement had to be found. And that other arrangement was to be the Superintendents' Society.[11]

Darche's comparative perspective also shed light on the plan for setting up a wider membership organization. By drawing out the precise ways in which the system of nurse training borrowed from Nightingale was altered to fit the United States, she was able to imply that these alterations themselves pointed to the need for a membership organization. At St. Thomas's Hospital the nurse trained for one year, then spent three years or more in hospitals. In America the nurse trained for two years, the first as a learner, the second in a responsible post in the hospital. Thereafter she went into practice in the community as a graduate nurse. From here, then, it was a short step to start considering devices for association and support, ways of aiding the isolated graduate nurse.

Nightingale's image of the trained nurse was of the hospital matron; the American leaders were always prone to think of the private nurse in the community.

Darche's comparison was perceptive and sensitive, but there was something curious about it. Darche had chosen to refer to a system that was by now thirty years old. For reasons that will become apparent, it is quite implausible to suggest that American nurses were ignorant of developments in Britain; what they were doing was apparently averting their gaze. A discreet veil was being cast over events in Britain and to understand the American strategy further it will help to raise the veil a little and glimpse inside.

Like the events of 1893 in the United States, the opening of St. Thomas's Hospital Nursing School had marked the arrival of a professionalizing strategy. It was more than a reform of nursing in a single setting, it was a deliberate plan to change the pattern of nursing in the hospitals. Darche, as we have seen, acknowledged this. She pointed out that the plan involved sending teams from St. Thomas's to nurse elsewhere. She was also clear that the plan was facilitated by pupils' loyalty to the Nightingale Fund and their willingness to be sent wherever the trustees suggested. The plan was aided by other factors too: by the respect and influence Nightingale had won as a result of her own activities, by the contacts she had as a result of her social position (which she was never slow to use), and by her having a small independent income. But the plan nonetheless posed problems.

In the first place, though Nightingale nurses spread widely and probably had an influence out of proportion to their numbers, the plan could not hope to transform the whole of hospital nursing. It proceeded, in fact, in parallel with nursing reforms of varying types in other hospitals. Second, the plan largely ignored the private nurse practicing in the community and the competition she faced from the untrained and disreputable, if she was a bona fide trained nurse. Third, and perhaps most important, it was a highly personal strategy. From her sickroom, Nightingale maintained close control and detailed contact with her nurses. The strategy required intense and unquestioning loyalty to a single, charismatic figure; it was, hence, unstable as well as limited in its reach.[12]

By the 1890s tension had begun to grow. While Nightingale herself saw no need for any kind of association of nurses beyond the link each nurse had with her own training school, and no way of judging the quality of a nurse except by personal knowledge of her, others had different views. Ethel Bedford Fenwick is of particular importance here and can be seen in some ways as responding directly to the weaknesses in the Nightingale strategy.[13]

Without a clearly recognized credential, the trained nurse outside the hospital was in an unhappy position. She could be undercut by the untrained nurse and her reputation could be diminished by the unsavory behavior of some who posed as nurses. Even in the hospital, trained nurses suffered when hospital authorities chose to appoint an untrained matron over them. Furthermore, the standards of some hospitals were appallingly low as far as nurse training was concerned. Bedford Fenwick's twin aims of distinguishing firmly the trained and untrained and of upgrading nurses flowed from these concerns. They led her toward highly controversial recommendations for registration of nurses, for closure of nursing to the untrained, and for specified educational entry requirements. Not only did these bring her into conflict with the system established by Nightingale, but they also provoked alarm among many practicing nurses and generated ire from hospital managements too. In short, hers was a quite different professionalizing strategy from Nightingale's and one that raised antagonisms in a variety of groups.[14]

By the time of the Chicago meeting Bedford Fenwick had already taken a number of important steps toward realizing her goals and had faced considerable obstacles. The British Nurses' Association (BNA), a body she was instrumental in creating, was by now six years old. It had tried, without success, to interest hospitals in forming boards to organize nurse education and to adhere to national standards. It had gained some medical support for the notion of a statutory register of nurses, only to find this route blocked by the maneuvers of opposing parties. In the summer of 1893 it gained a Royal Charter, under the terms of which the association itself could compile and maintain a register. But feelings were running high. Not only was Nightingale doing all that she could to subvert the BNA, but strenuous opposition was coming from the Hospitals' Association. Bedford Fenwick waged for many years a running battle with its spokesman, Sir Henry Burdett. Furthermore, that redoubtable lady was already perhaps ruminating, on that long sea voyage, on traitors within. For the very next year Bedford Fenwick and her doctor husband were to abandon the BNA and to pursue the battle for state registration through other means.

If the American nurses knew about all this, it can have held little allure for them. Lavinia Dock, who was later to build up a close knowledge of the international nursing scene and to visit London on a number of occasions and work with Bedford Fenwick, was to point out in 1905 that the troubles of British nurses were much greater than those of their

American counterparts. And Adelaide Nutting was later to confess that she had abandoned a plan to write a book on Florence Nightingale, given the "hornet's nest" of nursing matters in England. Bedford Fenwick would not have been slow to put her case in 1893 and certainly she had time to do it. She arrived early to superintend a display of British women's work and was treated as an "honoured guest," taking the opportunity of visiting American hospitals and doubtless of putting her views to her American colleagues while she did so.[15]

What the American nurses made of these views was another matter. Bedford Fenwick did not openly criticize Nightingale, but it was plain for all to see that the two women were at variance. What is more, her anger at Burdett and the Hospitals' Association was always open and vehement. Obviously the British situation was a delicate one. Our present state of knowledge of the parties involved leaves many questions open, but it does seem plausible that American nurses sought to avoid controversy and to avert repetition of the British pattern in their own country. Perhaps, then, this explains their emphasis on the establishment of a Superintendents' Society and the hesitation in discussing anything in detail beyond that. Britain, for them and in this respect, was not a model but a cautionary tale.[16]

From the foregoing, one can begin to see how a professionalizing strategy was woven together by American nurses. It was an active process in the sense that it involved much discussion and planning. But it was active also in that it involved a struggle to understand the past and the present as it affected nursing and a call upon external comparisons to help this process. Nurses were struggling here for insight into their own society and into how they might better adapt to and work within it. This struggle was producing a professional ideology—not just in the sense of a statement about the worth of their own occupational activity but in the broader sense of an understanding of the social division of labor in health care of which they were part. From that ideology, as influenced by its setting, a professionalizing strategy had begun to flow.

The British comparison, however, serves to point up features of the American strategy that its proponents took for granted. For one thing, the early organizations of nurses in Britain were built in conjunction with other parties, namely, the doctors and the hospital managers. Only later did British nurses organize on their own. In the United States there was no hint of this, and the organizations proposed were nurse organizations. For another thing, the key activity to promote change was different; in Britain the emphasis was on overt political action—to legislate or not to legislate was the dominant question. Legislation, of course, did come in the United States, but it came at the state not the federal level and it came as one plank in what Dock described firmly as an "educational movement"—somewhat mystifying the gentlemen of Britain's Select Committee on the Registration of Nurses, incidentally, who understood neither the educational improvement emphasis nor the strange practice of constantly amending state laws.[17]

There is a further contrast in that social differences were emphasized in British nursing organizations; it was the elite who organized—the well-born ladies educated at the London teaching hospitals—and they used their connections with the gentry to further their cause. Janet Wilson James has drawn attention to Lavinia Dock's observation about the cavalier exclusiveness of the original Superintendents' Society, but much depends on your point of comparison. What is striking to this British observer is the point that American nurses, simultaneously with setting up the Superintendents' Society, saw fit to give reassurances about an inclusive membership organization that would be run on democratic lines. But most striking of all is the American nurses' self-consciousness, their deliberate search to understand, their "stock-taking," and their institution-building.[18]

STRATEGY IN PERSPECTIVE

A final set of questions remains, questions that need to be asked in order to locate American nurses more firmly in their social setting. The "stock-taking" character of the events of 1893 is of the essence here, for this was no unique feature of American nursing. Its history is peppered with periods of self-analysis and review in a way that British nursing history is not—at least until recently. How may one account for the difference?[19]

The writings of an older generation of historians would appear to have relevance, particularly the concerns of those historians who have dealt with America as a new nation, lacking traditions and standing in an uneasy relationship to the traditions of the societies from which Americans have come. Daniel Boorstin long ago argued for the uniqueness of the American setting and institutions. Louis Hartz regarded the United States as a "fragment" society, suggesting that, in comprising mere fragments of other cultures, it necessarily could not embody any total pattern and was thus forced to develop along different lines. Seymour Martin Lipset, writing from a more sociological point of view, placed considerable emphasis on the revolutionary and colonial origins of the

United States and the values that stemmed from this. He argued that there were pressures to adapt institutions to these distinctive value patterns. Bernard Bailyn suggested that the institutional structure supporting European society was severely damaged in the course of transplantation, arguing that "on almost every major point the original inheritance was called into question, challenged by circumstances, altered or discarded." Bailyn's focus was on the family and formal education institutions. But we might well try to extend to occupational groups his speculation that a pattern that could remain unarticulated in the old setting became a conscious matter in the new, something for decision, will, and effort.[20]

The distinctiveness of American culture and values, while questioned by some scholars today, has been noted at least since the days of Alexis de Tocqueville, and it has been commented upon by sociologists and historians, using a wide variety of methodological and theoretical frameworks, no less than by foreign visitors. In all these works, the individualism of Americans is stressed, their emphasis on independence and on material gain, their belief in equality and achievement and in the openness of mobility prospects, their localism and disdain for governmental regulation. Is there, then, a direct congruence of values here? The Superintendents' Society was certainly a device that rested on ideas of individual freedom and perfectibility rather than on any notion of difference of interests and structural impediments to change. The idea of a membership organization, a voluntary association, further underlined self-help principles, which in no way involved imposing measures from a group above be it government or class.[21]

While professional ideologies may build upon and relate to broader societal values, there is, of course, more to it than that. Few writers today would be prepared to treat "values" or "culture" or "character" as a deus ex machina in the way that earlier analysts were prepared to do. Nor is it acceptable, as this paper has shown, to regard individuals and groups as entirely passive in their acceptance and reproduction of these social phenomena. The task, then, is to explore a matrix of values, situating them in their economic context, together with their associated political and social forms, and to ask what opportunities these offer for an occupationally organized group to form some kind of consciousness of itself as a collectivity and to take strategic actions of various sorts.

A hint of how this might be done may be found in the work of Robert Wiebe. He argues that the period around the turn of the century in the United States was one in which economic transformations had meant the breakup of isolated communities and the creation of a new urban order. The specialized needs of the urban populace were a "godsend" to professions, which began to shake off their old associations with the rich and privileged and to forge a new ideological base in the notion of functional skills. The development of groups such as doctors, lawyers, and teachers, Wiebe links with Progressivism and sees as integral to a new challenge and an emerging shift in the pattern of stratification. Arguments like these provide an interesting and suggestive framework in which to view more detailed work on the formation of professions in this period. Furthermore, Wiebe offers some comment on the position of women in all this: by working within tacit and mutually acceptable limits of women's concerns (social work and teaching are his examples), a select group of women were able to achieve a "smooth arrival" into the newly forming social order.[22]

How all this might compare with Britain is an interesting question. Recent work on medical practitioners seems to suggest that the struggle to achieve recognition for expertise dates from further back in the nineteenth century and is not firmly separated from older sources of power and authority until well into the twentieth century. Perhaps the concepts of the distinctive institutions of the "achieving society" (United States) versus the "open aristocracy" (Britain) still have an important heuristic value. However that may be, and while our understanding of the position of women and the nature of the women's movements in the two countries needs to be further developed and better integrated into even such suggestive works as Wiebe's, it is Wiebe's interpretation of the early twentieth century that begins to provide a time-specific framework that is helpful in making sense of the developments with which I have been concerned.[23]

By focusing on a rather small segment of American nursing history and relating the data thus revealed to developments in Britain, to general interpretations of American culture and values, and to a specific interpretation of the era under consideration, I hope to have shown the value of disaggregating the broad and ambiguous concept of professionalization into such smaller and more precise concepts as professionalizing strategy and professional ideology. Coupled to the kind of cross-cultural comparative investigation I have undertaken, concepts such as these are still flexible enough to help us to recover the nuances and complexities of nurse organization in different countries, and to dislodge the general tendency to portray occupations as though they occupied some timeless mid-Atlantic space. American nurses traveled the Atlantic, both literally and metaphorically; and they were active in their efforts to make sense of their experiences and to profit from them.

NOTES

The research on which this paper is based was carried out with the aid of a United Kingdom Social Science Research Council grant (HR 4465). I would like to acknowledge the help and support of Professor Margaret Stacey throughout the project. An earlier version of this paper was presented at the British Sociological Association, Medical Sociology Section Conference, York, September 1978. Thanks for comments should go to Robert Dingwall, John Ehrenreich, Dag Hofoss, and Margaret Stacey.

1. The text of Toner's speech is reprinted as it appeared in the *Evening Star* in Dorothy J. Youtz, *The Capital City School of Nursing* (Washington, D.C.: Capital City School of Nursing Alumnae, 1975), pp. 27–28.

2. For information on these various visits and visitors, see Dorothy Giles, *A Candle in Her Hand: A Story of the Nursing Schools of Bellevue Hospital* (New York: G. P. Putnam's Sons, 1949); Ethel Johns and Blanche Pfefferkorn, *The Johns Hopkins Hospital School of Nursing 1889–1949* (Baltimore: Johns Hopkins University Press, 1954); and Janet Wilson James, "Isabel Hampton and the Professionalization of Nursing in the 1880s," in *The Therapeutic Revolution: Essays in the Social History of American Medicine*, ed. Charles E. Rosenberg and Morris J. Vogel (Philadelphia: University of Pennsylvania Press, 1979), pp. 201–44. For an interesting recent study of the influence of one British nurse working in the United States, see Nancy Tomes, " 'Little World of Our Own': The Pennsylvania Hospital Training School for Nurses, 1895–1907," *Journal of the History of Medicine and Allied Sciences* 33 (1978): 507–30.

3. For examples of the approach to professionalization that posits a fixed sequence of events, see Theodore Caplow, *The Sociology of Work* (Minneapolis: University of Minnesota Press, 1954) and Harold Wilensky, "The Professionalization of Everyone," *American Journal of Sociology* 70 (1964): 137–58; for early statements of the view that professionalization is "about power," see Eliot Friedson, *Profession of Medicine: A Study of the Sociology of Applied Knowledge* (New York: Harper & Row, 1970) and Terence Johnson, *Professions and Power* (London: Macmillan, 1942). A fuller discussion of this, dealing especially with difficulties in the "power" model of professionalization can be found in Celia Davies, "Professional Power & Sociological Analysis: Lessons from a Comparative Historical Study of Nursing in Britain and the U.S.A." (Ph.D. dissertation, University of Warwick, 1981).

4. Some might still want to say that there is nothing distinctly "professional" in these definitions, and why not therefore refer to occupational ideology and occupational strategy. This may well be right. We need to make comparative studies of ideologies and strategies among those who call them-

selves professional and those who do not to see to what extent and in what direction ideologies as well as strategies are articulated.

5. The account of the Chicago meeting, which follows, may be compared with that of James, "Isabel Hampton." My account, written originally in 1978, relied largely on the papers reprinted in Isabel Hampton et al., *Nursing of the Sick—1893* (New York: McGraw-Hill, 1949). James's account is based on a wider range of sources and is concerned with matters beyond professional strategy as defined here. There are a few points of disagreement, however, and where there are, I draw attention to them.

6. Hampton, *Nursing of the Sick*, pp. 157–58; see also Lavinia L. Dock, *A History of Nursing*, 4 vols. (New York: G. P. Putnam's Sons, 1912), vol. 3; Helen E. Marshall, *Mary Adelaide Nutting: Pioneer of Modern Nursing* (Baltimore: Johns Hopkins University Press, 1972).

7. The papers by McIsaac, Draper, and Sutcliffe can all be found reprinted in Hampton, *Nursing of the Sick*. It is interesting to note in connection with Sutcliffe that James, "Isabel Hampton," describes her as clinging to the Nightingale image. Another factor accounting for her comment and for the fear of associations as degrading could well have been the link in nurses' minds with labor unrest and with trade unions. I am grateful to John Ehrenreich for pointing this out to me.

8. Celia Davies, "Making Sense of the Census in Britain and the U.S.A.: The Changing Occupational Classification and the Position of Nurses," *Sociological Review* 28 (1980): 581–609.

9. For work that deals with the economic factors involved in nurse training, see Jo Ann Ashley, *Hospitals, Paternalism, and the Role of the Nurse* (New York: Teachers College Press, 1976); Susan Reverby, "The Search for the Hospital Yardstick: Nursing and the Rationalization of Hospital Work," in *Health Care in America: Essays in Social History*, ed. Susan Reverby and David Rosner (Philadelphia: Temple University Press, 1979), pp. 206–25; and Celia Davies, "A Constant Casualty: Nurse Education in Britain and the U.S.A. to 1939," in *Rewriting Nursing History*, ed. Celia Davies (London: Croom Helm, 1980) pp. 102–22. The quotation is from Hampton, *Nursing of the Sick*, p. 8.

10. Ibid., p. 10. For a discussion of "progress" in nursing history, see Celia Davies, "The Contemporary Challenge in Nursing History," in *Rewriting Nursing History*, pp. 11–17.

11. For the Darche quotations, see her address in Hampton, *Nursing of the Sick*, p. 98.

12. For information on Nightingale nurses, see Lucy R. Seymer, *Florence Nightingale's Nurses: The Nightingale Training School, 1860–1960* (London: Pitman Medical Publishing, 1960). For accounts of other hospital reforms and schools, see Sarah Tooley, *The History of Nursing in the British Empire* (London: Bousfield, 1906).

13. Ethel Bedford Fenwick (née Manson) was matron of St. Bar-

tholomew's Hospital from 1881 to 1887. After her marriage to Dr. Bedford Fenwick she continued to be active in nursing, being influential in the formation of a number of important associations and expressing her opinions forcibly as editor of the *Nursing Record*. Her aggressive manner seems to have given her a bad press. Brian Abel-Smith, *A History of the Nursing Profession* (London: Heinemann, 1960), on whose detailed account I have relied here, is nonetheless remarkably unsympathetic, and although Winifred Hector, *The Work of Mrs. Bedford Fenwick & the Rise of Professional Nursing* (London: Royal College of Nursing, 1973) does something to retrieve the situation, more work is needed on this key figure. Her relation to feminist ideas and her position in relation to medicine are topics that need particular investigation.

14.   Abel Smith, *History of the Nursing Profession*, brings these conflicts out very clearly.

15.   For Dock's comparison, see Lavinia Dock, "The Progress of Registration," *American Journal of Nursing* 5 (1905–6): 297–305. Marshall, *Mary Adelaide Nutting*, gives several hints of Nutting's links to British nursing, and Hector, *The Work of Mrs. Bedford Fenwick*, deals with Bedford Fenwick's visit to the United States.

16.   James, "Isabel Hampton," has suggested that Hampton and Dock were disappointed at Draper's tentative paper on the "Necessity for an American Nurses' Association"; Dock, *History of Nursing*, reports that it was Hampton's most cherished vision and that she had poured forth her hopes about it in a letter to Draper. So it seems, not surprisingly, that there were divisions also within American nursing.

17.   This comes over clearly in the verbatim record of the cross-examination of Dock and the way in which her questioners keep coming back to the point that the registration is permissive and not compulsory. Finally she did agree that compulsion might help. See Select Committee on the Registration of Nurses, *Minutes of Evidence* (1905), paragraphs 777–839.

18.   James, "Isabel Hampton," p. 231.

19.   Davies, "Professional Power" and "A Constant Casualty," deal with the differences in self-consciousness between British and American nurses.

20.   Daniel J. Boorstin, *The Americans*, 3 vols. (New York: Random House, 1958–73); Louis Hartz, *The Founding of New Societies* (New York: Harcourt, Brace & World, 1964); Seymour Martin Lipset, *The First New Nation* (New York: Basic Books, 1963); and Bernard Bailyn, *Education in the Forming of American Society* (Chapel Hill: University of North Carolina Press, 1960). The quotation from Bailyn is from p. 48.

21.   See Johan Huizinga, *America: A Dutch Historian's Vision from Afar and Near* (New York: Harper & Row, 1972); Richard Hofstadter and Seymour Martin Lipset, eds., *Turner and the Sociology of the Frontier* (New York: Basic Books, 1968); and John Lankford, "The Writing of American

History in the 1960s: A Critical Bibliography of Interest to Sociologists," *Sociological Quarterly* 14 (1973): 99–126.

22. Robert H. Wiebe, *The Search for Order, 1877–1920* (New York: Hill & Wang, 1967). See also Corinne L. Gilb, *Hidden Hierarchies: The Professions and Government* (New York: Harper & Row, 1966).

23. On the British medical profession, see M. Jeanne Peterson, *The Medical Profession in Mid-Victorian London* (Berkeley: University of California Press, 1978). The term "open aristocracy" is drawn from the work of the British social historian Harold Perkin, *The Origins of Modern English Society 1780–1880* (London: Routledge & Kegan Paul, 1969). There are some historical discussions of the professions in the British social structure, but not many. See A. M. Carr-Saunders and P. A. Wilson, *The Professions* (Oxford: Clarendon Press, 1933) and W. J. Reader, *Professional Men: The Rise of the Professional Classes in Nineteenth Century England* (London: Weidenfeld & Nicolson, 1966). For one suggestion of a comparative historical approach, see Michael Burrage, "The Group Ties of Occupations in Britain and the United States," *Administrative Science Quarterly* 17 (1972): 240–53. I do not mean to imply in the discussion above that there is no comparative work on the women's movement in Britain and the United States, which, of course, there is. Rather, I am suggesting that it is still difficult to follow up leads such as the one that British nursing was more class-divided than American nursing. For what there is on that, see Abel-Smith, *History of the Nursing Profession*; Michael Carpenter, "The New Managerialism and Professionalism in Nursing," in *Health Care and the Division of Labour*, ed. Margaret Stacey, et al. (London: Croom Helm, 1977); and M. Adelaide Nutting and Lavinia Dock, *A History of Nursing* (New York: G. P. Putnam's Sons, 1907), pp. 385–86.

4

Public Health, Midwives, and Nurses, 1880–1930

Jane Pacht Brickman

I

Some recent analysts of contemporary American obstetrics have expressed outrage at the "undue" medical orientation of childbirth. For these authors obstetrics represents the culmination of male usurpation of the traditional female role as birth attendant. Moreover, male professional supremacy carries a regrettable corollary—female passivity. Viewed historically, contemporary critics have argued, the hospital's replacement of the home as the place for birth heaped indignities upon women. Many became victims of irrational institutional procedures, which threatened essential bonding between mother and newborn. Hospitalization also depersonalized a central experience in women's lives, once rich in family ritual and closeness. More unpardonable still, institutional confinement facilitated an escalation of technical interference. In hospitals, doctors subjected women to elective labor induction, routine employment of analgesics and anesthesia, and episiotomies. Resort to forceps and Caesarean section rose precipitously, as did the vague and dubious indications for these procedures. Indeed, the very fatalities that obstetricians used to justify their ascendancy often resulted from these interventions. Instead of becoming safer, childbirth presented a key arena for iatrogenic disease and death.[1]

Directly and indirectly, recent critics of childbirth practices have raised new issues about late nineteenth- and early twentieth-century transitions in maternal health care. In particular they have posed new questions concerning the elimination of the midwife. Midwifery mushroomed in the first third of the twentieth century, largely as a result of European immigrations, yet later slipped into precipitous decline. The contraction certainly related to attacks by physicians, whose criticisms of midwives' cleanliness, integrity, and abilities amounted to a scare campaign to corrode women's confidence in the naturalness of childbirth. By exaggerating their own omnipotence, as well as the pathology of pregnancy and delivery, doctors could assert their superior expertise.

Some historians have found gender hostility at the root of medical opposition to the midwife. They have contended that the midwife's elimination in America resulted from subtle sexist assumptions about female incapacities for technical mastery and from outright misogyny.[2]

But these explanations prove too simple. For one thing, European obstetrics continues to rely upon the midwife; yet male attitudes across the Atlantic are undoubtedly no different. Furthermore, had American midwives been the victims of male doctors' unwillingness to share their profession across gender lines, women doctors presumably would have championed their cause. That never happened. More important, however, to assume that the midwife's failure to survive the immigrants' voyage from Europe resulted from male hostility disconnects the "midwife debate" from other contemporary health-related issues. These included questions of professionalization of health-care groups and their place in the delivery network, the provision of care for the indigent and working classes, the value of preventive medicine, and whether the risks of accidents and illness should be shared. Stressing sexism as a primary factor in the male hegemony of medicine, or obstetrics, ignores the issues of power, status, and economics that preoccupied the medical profession during the early part of the twentieth century.[3]

For these reasons this paper posits an alternative interpretation. It argues that midwives might have formed an indispensable part of our health apparatus, if their survival had not been incompatible with the so-called therapeutic revolution in medicine and a fee-for-service, profit-making system. It urges that the elimination of the midwife had little to do with either the gender or the capacities of these female birth attendants. Far more important were the struggles of the medical profession to define itself as an elite body with layers of specialties, and the inadequacies of the public health movement. These elements, in combination, made the elimination of the midwife almost inevitable, even though contemporary studies demonstrated that midwives' attendance at normal childbirth was safer and more aseptic than delivery by most physicians still engaged in home birth.[4]

This does not suggest that doctors consciously connived the downfall of midwives in the service of their bank accounts. At the turn of the century, articulate medical spokesmen had two primary concerns. First, they sought a general improvement in American health standards. They hoped to challenge high rates of disease and death with the promises offered by the universal application of modern medical technology and the germ theory. Second, they endeavored to set their house in order—to unify the profession to assure members both public acknowledgment and financial certainty. When doctors urged the replacement of midwives with medical specialists, they undoubtedly believed they were serving the public by substituting scientifically trained personnel for lay people; midwives' truncated education and more casual approach to obstetrics conflicted with the new image of medical expertise. Midwives' practices certainly contradicted new medical norms, but this was not all. They threatened American Medical Association (AMA) efforts for professional homogenization, designed to extirpate divisive nineteenth-century elements of a multiplicity of practitioners, educational standards, and fee scales, which had been so detrimental to professional prestige and practice.

The venue and circumstances of her practice also colored medical attitudes toward the midwife. If she were to conform to modern medical knowledge, she would have to come under public supervision, often as a salaried employee in a public clinic. Her survival would necessarily strengthen the public sector of medicine, and the controversy her presence stirred linked itself to the wider AMA effort to deliver health care in a privately controlled and unregulated market.

II

As many scholars have noted, the early decades of the twentieth century saw pivotal changes in the history of the American medical profession. Throughout the nineteenth century, competing sects of healers had vied for public recognition and support and for the financial rewards of medical practice. At the end of the nineteenth century, allopathic or "regular" physicians, institutionally represented by the AMA (established in 1847 to represent them), made peace with homeopaths and eclectics. Doctors had achieved enough cohesion so that state authorities could establish licensing boards, with members from each of the three schools. Having closed the door to fringe practitioners and paved the way for professional unity, the medical leadership could now focus on what it perceived as a glut of practitioners.[5]

Led by the AMA's Council on Medical Education, formed in 1904, leaders in the profession began to work for the elimination of "inferior" medical schools and the adoption of stiffer entrance and graduation requirements at the "superior" ones. By raising "standards," practitioners could limit the number of medical graduates. Hence just as the nineteenth century had sprouted medical schools, the twentieth century squashed them. Schools began to close around 1906, and the trend received powerful reinforcement from the publication of Abraham Flexner's 1910 report on medical education.[6]

Plagued throughout the nineteenth century with sectarian divisions, the medical profession began to coalesce just as turn-of-the-century waves of European immigration brought an unexpected revival of midwifery. The profession, sensitive to invasions of its territory, found the resurgence threatening. Moreover, midwives' presence posed a special challenge to a particularly vulnerable specialty within medicine.

Early in the twentieth century, obstetrics was still characterized as the "pot boiler of the profession, the chief resource of the young and inexperienced and least trained physician, to be abandoned as soon as possible for a less arduous and rest-disturbing and more remunerative field." Traditionally, obstetrical services had been little more than an opening wedge through which a general practitioner sought and won a clientele. A calculating physician would take on childbirth in the hope of winning confidence and with that the more lucrative family practice. As midwifery expanded, doctors' opportunities diminished. Stark reality showed that "some 30,000 women have taken enough practice away from the physician to obtain livelihood." Yet increasingly the struggle against the midwife represented obstetricians' efforts to wrest childbirth from the hands of the medical generalist and the midwife alike. With the obstetrical specialist aspiring to independent recognition within the medical world, the midwife as well as the general practitioner delivering babies at home could undermine his claim that childbirth belonged in the hospital.[7]

For the obstetrician the presence in New York City in 1915 of a "body of 1,448 midwives [who] deliver approximately 53,000 babies per year, [while] all that the lying-in hospitals . . . can care for is 11,000" proved a call to action. If specialists could convince the public of their indispensability, the imbalance would be corrected. Early twentieth-century medical appraisals rather abruptly made pregnancy, labor, and delivery pathological risks. Reliance on midwives would perpetuate the undesirable view "that human reproduction is a normal physiological process. This may have been true in prehistoric times," spokesmen for a prominent New York City maternity hospital asserted, but "it is not true now." According to physicians, midwives were incapable of recognizing the frequent abnormalities of labor. Further, proper prenatal care, with blood pressure readings and urinalysis, lay beyond the midwife's scope, as did adequate medical inspection of the newborn.[8]

According to physicians, midwives posed more than theoretical risks, and bore responsibility for the frequent gynecological surgery following unmended childbirth lacerations, and for the prevalence of blindness from ophthalmia neonatorum (caused by gonorrheal bacteria, which the infant contracts in passage through the birth canal). In 1907 one physician even blamed midwives for one-third of the abortions in New York City. His charge may or may not have been just, but having failed to consider the responsibility of doctors in the remaining known cases, this commentator revealed an agenda he shared with many of his colleagues. By denigrating the competence of midwives, obstetricians reinforced arguments for the services they could uniquely provide: anesthesia (and particularly twilight sleep, a twentieth-century invention), version, forceps, and Caesarean section. These procedures required a hospital setting, and effectively excluded both the general practitioner and the midwife.[9]

Quite possibly by the early twentieth century physicians could not imagine good obstetrical care without optional recourse to forceps and chloroform. Certainly these medical advances gave childbirth the potential for greater safety and comfort. Categorical censorship of midwifery practice may have stemmed partially from a new professional perspective, which viewed the withholding of life-saving techniques as criminally negligent. For these reasons many doctors may have believed "that no training under the sun could make her [the midwife] a competent obstetrical attendant."[10]

Yet some physicians understood and conceded that the midwife's European training was "far superior" to the education "the great majority of physicians receive in this country before graduation," and that the German midwife's oral and written examination "is one that the average graduate of an American medical school would have difficulty in passing with distinction." Still, these doctors dismissed European training paradigms as irrelevant to circumstances in the United States. They were expensive and would foster resentment among licensed physicians.[11]

It is difficult to avoid the conclusion that obstetricians feared that more than all the purported hazards that the midwife posed to her patients, giving the midwife a distinct place would sink the physician's position. With six months' training, women could be doctors' equals for most cases. Supervision of the midwife would create two obstetrical standards, which was considered an intolerable situation. Having long remained in an ambivalent position themselves, obstetricians saw the midwife's sudden flourishing as a drag on their professional progress. "As long as the medical profession tolerates that brand of infamy, the midwife," one physician remarked, "the public will not be brought to realize that there is a high art in obstetrics and that it must pay as well for it as for surgery." Without a uniform obstetrical standard, "the modern tendency . . . to lift obstetrics to the level of medicine and surgery" seemed impossible.[12]

The alternative was clear. Specialists recommended educating the public to recognize "such a thing as the 'science and art of obstetrics,'" rather than training the midwife. They sought to educate the public to the nature of the obstetrician's skill, "so time and strength-consuming, and so exacting," in order to increase willingness "to duly compensate him for the work." Recognition of the midwife, they warned, would demoralize the profession. How could the medical student be convinced to "specialize [in obstetrics] when midwives and practitioners deliver babies without training"?[13]

III

Medical animus against the midwife focused on the urban practitioner, whose resurgence flowed from strong preferences among immigrant mothers. Wherever immigrants settled, the midwife flourished. Newcomers shunned the hospital, which tended to be remote from most foreign residential enclaves and alien in language. Moreover, birth often afforded the occasion for festive celebration (the Jewish custom of circumcision, for example) which required the woman and child to be at home. The midwife, almost always foreign born and living in the community, lay in the buffer that immigrant groups maintained against an already overwhelming cultural shock.[14]

Equally important, with the hospital (for the rich or charity patient) and the private physician (usually a general practitioner with no obstetric expertise) as the only alternatives to midwife delivery, the midwife became an economic necessity. She charged less and did more.

As part of the social network of relationships in immigrant ghettos, the midwife served as woman's confidante, offering herbal remedies for female ills as well as abortions. She stood by the woman through labor and returned to the home for postpartum care, from five to ten days after birth. In the home the midwife performed household services, cooking, cleaning, and supervising children, for which she charged between $7.00 and $10.00. Simple delivery care by a physician, with no postpartum observation, cost between $20.00 and $25.00.[15]

Custom and economics aside, the immigrant had a strong rational foundation for her preference, based upon midwives' capabilities in Europe. There, where governments licensed and supervised all midwives, training ranged from a six-month program in official health clinics in Germany to a year's instruction in Norway, Sweden, Denmark, and Britain and two years of courses in Holland, France, and Belgium. The European midwife could not legally practice without training, and governments tested competency periodically. Midwives attended 75 percent of all deliveries in England in the mid-1920s, and the country's maternal mortality remained lower than in the United States.[16]

Immigrant preference for the midwife could have been supported if, as in Europe, American jurisdictions had legitimated her role with regulation or education. Under American laissez-faire conditions, however, the midwife remained a declassed person. This obviously facilitated her ultimate demise. In the few places that sought to duplicate the ubiquitous European regulatory schemes (individual cities such as New York, Newark, and Philadelphia; statewide in New York, New Jersey, Connecticut, Pennsylvania), expedience ruled. Most public health leaders urged midwifery regulation, but only as a temporary measure. While attempts to elevate standards were sincere, health administrators rarely saw the midwife as more than a necessary—and most likely ephemeral—evil.[17]

Public health officials might concede that "theoretically the midwife should not exist," but they admitted that immediate abolition was unrealistic. In 1915 Dr. Linsly Williams, New York State deputy commissioner of health, noted that outside of New York City, midwives reported a fourth of all births in the state. Abolishing the midwife without substitutes would mean "either that midwives would continue to practice without a license, or that their patients would not be able to receive any assistance whatsoever during the period of childbirth."[18]

Public health leaders suggested educational programs for the existing midwife population, with simultaneous increases in free public health facilities. Health reformers viewed regulation as safety protection, not as an "attempt to perpetuate [midwifery] as a separate profession." New indoor (hospital ward) and outdoor (outpatient ambulatory) facilities would slowly draw poor women from the midwife.[19]

Dual and contradictory goals hampered health reformers' efforts to widen the base of medical care. Public health activists, building upon the nucleus of dispensary organization, established America's first community health centers. And yet, however much health advocates succeeded in spreading the benefits of modern medicine across class lines, the innovations they championed proved as susceptible to the "progressive" faith in efficiency and expertise as most of their generation. Midwives, however capable or willing to cooperate in pilot projects, did not qualify as "experts" and could not fit reformers' constructs of disinterested technicians bringing order to the chaos of industrial and urban society.[20]

Health activists bypassed the midwife in their efforts to bring better obstetrical care to poor women, trusting instead the medical profession. Public health officials sought to make the midwife a safe attendant and included her in prenatal centers, but only as a stopgap to be replaced by medical personnel. Fearful of alienating immigrants and aware that the midwife attracted foreign-born women to health demonstrations, prenatal workers claimed that they neither "discriminated against the midwife nor promoted her welfare." But workers for the New York Milk Committee, a voluntary health agency promoting preventive baby care, signaled their acceptance of physicians' "expertise" by urging medical confinement whenever possible. As they put it:

> Whenever we could tactfully do so . . . we advised the employment of a physician at confinement. If the financial conditions of the home were such as to prohibit this, the family was advised to go to a hospital or take advantage of the free out-patient department of the Maternity Hospitals [sic]. Where cases had engaged midwives, no effort was made to discourage their plan. Where the mother seemed determined to employ a midwife the Bellevue School of Midwives was suggested.[21]

Even where midwifery supervision reflected a respect for immigrant tastes, municipal regulation reduced the number of active midwives and fed into obstetricians' unrelenting desires to drive off competition. In New York City, for example, 3,191 midwives practiced in 1909, reporting attendance at 49,616 births, or 40 percent of the total; in 1920, after twelve years of licensing, the city roster carried only 1,517 practicing midwives who delivered 36,369 women in childbirth for 26 percent of the total. The downward trend accelerated. In 1923 midwives in the city delivered 21 percent of the births, and in 1933 midwives handled merely 8.5 percent of the deliveries.[22]

IV

Thus the historian confronts a paradox. Aware of a need for birth-related health care services and of immigrants' widespread willingness to turn to midwives for assistance, early twentieth-century health reformers refused to acknowledge midwives' real capacities and never tried to establish a distinct place for them within the health care system. Why not?

When educated, the midwife offered safe care, perhaps safer than doctors. When city departments regulated her, the midwife often established effective mutuality with health officials. Regulation seemed to inspire midwives' professional pride. When the system legitimated her distinct role, the midwife reciprocated. Physicians' hostile charges of midwives' stubbornness and individualism appear to have been mythical, clear fabrications without substance.

For example, after collaborating with the city's midwives and emphasizing the importance of prenatal care, the staff of the Division of Midwives and Foundlings of the New York City Bureau of Child Hygiene discovered that 65 percent of those receiving city prenatal care had enrolled upon midwives' referrals (substantially in excess of the proportion of women who actually used midwives for delivery). "Of this number," Dr. S. Josephine Baker, the bureau's head, reported in 1914, "we have had no deaths, no cases of ophthalmia neonatorum or eclampsia." In 1916, with about 40 percent of births in midwives' hands, only 22 percent of the city's deaths from puerperal sepsis could be traced to their deliveries. Physicians, who reported approximately 60 percent of the city's births, bore responsibility for 69 percent of deaths from puerperal septicemia.[23]

Many other observers also realized that supervised midwives posed no danger. In Providence, Rhode Island, where midwives worked with city officials, their infant mortality fell to 77 (per 1,000 live births) against a rate of 117 for the rest of the city. In Buffalo health workers reported that midwives' patients suffered significantly less operative interference, although midwives had called for medical aid when needed. In 1913 Newark's Division of Child Hygiene began working with the midwife. Capitalizing on the established influence of the midwife—they delivered 50 percent of the city's babies—district nurses relied on the midwife to service their prenatal clientele. Julius Levy, director of the division, felt more than satisfied. Maternal mortality in Newark dropped steadily, to compare favorably with other large cities. In 1914 it stood at 5.3 per 1,000 births; by 1915 the rate fell to 3.6 and in 1916 it was 2.2. In 1916 in Boston, where the midwife was illegal, the maternal mortality rate remained at 6.5.[24]

Did any data provide statistical validity for excluding the midwife? In the case of ophthalmia neonatorum, which caused seven thousand cases of blindness in the United States in 1910, studies failed to corroborate physicians' allegations. The prophylactic application of two drops of 1 percent solution of silver nitrate in each eye immediately upon birth easily prevented the infection. In 1909 the Massachusetts Eye and Ear Infirmary investigated 116 cases. In only two did midwives deliver the victims, while 114 came under doctors' care. This was not an isolated example. Nurses of the New York City Health Department visited the homes of twenty-seven cases of the infection and noted that in twenty-two, physicians had attended the births. The New York School of Philanthropy similarly sampled thirty-three cases of infant blindness and discovered that physicians had been responsible for the deliveries of twenty-two and midwives for eleven. Research by the Boston School of Social Work in five Massachusetts cities found doctors using lemon juice in place of silver nitrate; of the ninety-five doctors interviewed, only 17 percent routinely used the procedure. "It is common knowledge," wrote Jacob Sobel of the New York City Bureau of Child Hygiene, "that prophylactic instillation into the eyes of the newborn of various silver preparations is more commonly practiced by the midwives of this city than by physicians."[25]

In light of this, and the fact that some public health activists had statistical proof of the midwife's capabilities, why did they not crusade on her behalf, challenging medical resistance and physicians' rhetoric? Part of the answer lies in the choices that women themselves made, which encouraged health reformers to see the midwife's function as transitional and temporary at best. By the early twentieth century, wealthy women had already abandoned the midwife for the physician, and as immigrant daughters matured, many proved anxious to adopt American ways. Because the midwife carried the stigma of the premodern culture to which their mothers clung, some immigrants' daughters declined her services. Indeed, especially by the 1920s, many immigrants themselves, delivering second and third children, turned to the doctor and hospital. Particularly when the family economic situation improved, they discarded the midwife, now associated with ghetto life and public clinics. Finally the congressional restrictions on immigration in the 1920s posed significant barriers to sustained demand for midwives' services.

Yet the shift reflected far more than women's fickle tastes. Legitimating the midwife's work would have challenged the economic and social status of the medical profession, and, to some extent, the bacteriological approach to medical care. That midwives could provide services comparable to obstetricians' at a fraction of the fee belied specialists' claims. Moreover, midwives, unlike hospital nurses, were never subordinate to late nineteenth- and early twentieth-century physicians. Instead they occupied a collateral position. Midwives dealt independently with their clientele, and their outpatient, almost casual approach demystified childbirth, diminishing its content against the specialties of medicine and surgery.

Beyond that, midwives offered care that stressed indigenous and holistic qualities, again exemplifying an approach that had become anathema to the medical profession. Unlike obstetrics, midwifery was not organized around a pathological model. To have sanctioned midwifery would have been tantamount to questioning the validity of the germ theory of disease as the basis for all health care. Having endowed medical therapy with greater precision and heightened its "scientific" legitimacy, the germ theory proved vital to the medical profession's new self-definition and public image. For contemporaries, both private practitioner and reformer alike, midwives' practices might well have appeared irreconcilable with new forms of medical intervention creating nothing short of a health revolution. At the same time, the new methods elevated physicians' reputations and financial security.

The simultaneous flowering of health reform and medical consolidation became a final factor in the complex matrix of medical reactions to the midwife. Because the resurgence of midwifery occurred at the height of the early twentieth-century public health movement, organized medicine's opposition to the midwife meshed with its growing suspicion of public health reform in general. Indeed, organized medicine coalesced around the goal of professional unity just as urban ghetto conditions made it impossible to ignore poor people's health any longer. Physicians' battles to ensure status thus coincided with reformers' efforts to create a public health care system, requiring organized medicine to work not only for a homogeneous group of practitioners, but also to define the contours of modern medicine against the state.

The public health movement, although clearly part of early

twentieth-century liberal reform, challenged medical autonomy. In his presidential address to the 75th annual meeting of the AMA in Chicago in June 1924, William Allen Pusey summarized the perceived threat:

> There is an evident tendency now to appropriate medicine in the social movement; to make the treatment of the sick a function of society as a whole; to take it away from the individual's responsibilities and to transfer it to the state; to turn it over to organized movements.

Pusey's statement may have exaggerated the dimensions of the public health movement, but his views are important here because they illustrate the degree to which the medical struggle against the midwife, far from proceeding in isolation, was linked to the larger AMA effort to limit public health activity generally. Physicians' opposition to the midwife is therefore best understood as a complement to their contemporaneous battles against national health insurance and the Sheppard-Towner Act of 1921, which extended federal funds to the states for educational programs to promote welfare in maternity and infancy.[26]

Significantly, for example, when Dr. George W. Kosmak testified against the Sheppard-Towner bill in 1921, he restated a concern frequently voiced in discussions of the midwife: she threatened a return to the nineteenth-century healing tradition of multiple categories of independent practitioners. Ignoring objections ranging from allegations of fiscal extravagance to visions of communist conspiracy, Kosmak and the American Gynecological Society focused on more concrete matters. The bill seemed to portend lay usurpation of medical hegemony, he claimed. It seemed to threaten the subordination of medical therapy to sociological experiment administered by public health doctors, social workers, and visiting nurses. Working as peers, nonphysicians delivering health care could damage the physician's preeminence in the medical hierarchy.[27]

Speaking before a House of Representatives committee, in defense of the American Gynecological Society's resolution against the Sheppard-Towner bill, Kosmak said:

> We feel . . . that turning over such important matters into the hands of what we . . . consider lay people, will act to the discredit of the medical profession and also as a bar to its development. . . . [Today] there are scarcely 150,000 physicians. If by legislative enactment you are going to turn over an important part of their work into the hands of nurses . . . you will at once interpose

> a stumbling block to the progress of medicine, because young men
> will not compete under those circumstances with trained nurses.

Grounded in a century's insecurity, Kosmak's statement reflected the medical establishment's anxiety over its newly won monopolization of health care. With nurses (and others) assuming independent, rather than subordinate, roles in the medical network, both the pocketbook and the status of private physicians would be in jeopardy. Furthermore, because the public health nurse under Sheppard-Towner, like the midwife when regulated, would work under the umbrella of public supervision, the act raised the specter of government control of medicine and the loss of its free-enterprise spirit.[28]

Arguments against Sheppard-Towner tended to prophesy the doom of the fabric and integrity of the social order. But the act proved benign. Unlike health insurance which theoretically meant resource redistribution (albeit minimal), the Sheppard-Towner Act never touched upon the structure of American asset ownership, nor did it tell doctors how to practice. The act provided no substitute free care in hospitals or clinics, and never challenged the fee-for-service principle. It merely embodied the earliest tenet of the public health movement: the notion that wider dissemination of knowledge would narrow the cleavage between the haves and have-nots. Nevertheless opposition to Sheppard-Towner, and to the public health movement generally, illustrates why, from the point of view of organized medicine, the midwife had to die.[29]

V

To overcome organized medicine's hostility, public health officials would have had to defend the midwife in terms of a "public interest." But the retention of the midwife never became part of a national public health platform, as did pure milk, prenatal examinations, early immunization, and uniform criteria for medical specialists' certification. Only insistence by reformers, combined with municipal and state government intervention through educational and licensing requirements, might have saved the midwife from physicians' efforts to abolish her. Sporadic support proved insufficient, but that was all she got.

While some health leaders, notably Clara D. Noyes, Carolyn Van Blarcom, S. Josephine Baker, Grace Abbott, Jacob Sobel, and Julius Levy, came to view the midwife as a welcome ally in the battle against infant and maternal mortality, they never conceded that her distinct, paramedical function was intrinsic to the public's health. In a day of organization for the promotion of health issues, effective persuasion would have required that the midwife's defenders combine to urge her cause. Instead, and again at a time when activists joined regularly in concerted support of specific reform causes, to the extent that any championed the midwife, they did so as individuals.[30]

Some eminent public health spokesmen, like Abraham Jacobi, Mary Beard, and Mary Breckinridge, argued for midwives on the basis of their worth. Most often, however, proponents merely defended the midwife's record, and perhaps her possibilities in the context of an immigrant population, without arguing her potential for the future. Moreover, even public health advocates who promoted the midwife were at least as satisfied when women chose a physician for childbirth delivery. Jacob Sobel, a staunch defender of the midwife, echoed the statement of the New York Milk Committee when he described the typical procedures of New York City's Bureau of Child Hygiene:

> Mothers are always urged . . . to place themselves under medical care, but if they express preference for a midwife, they are referred to midwives who are known to be graduates of the recognized school of this city, the Bellevue Hospital School for Midwives.[31]

Similarly S. Josephine Baker recalled the "trouble" New York City's obstetricians made for the bureau when it began its program of regulating and training midwives. The obstetricians'

> [I]dea was that the best thing would be to stamp out midwifery altogether instead of compromising with it. The doctors were never able to understand the sort of people we had to deal with. If deprived of midwives, these women would rather have amateur assistance from the janitor's wife or the woman across the hall than submit to this outlandish American custom of having in a male doctor for a confinement. Their daughters, the second generation of mothers, were a different matter, and learned to insist upon employing doctors as any American girl.

Baker showed no regret at the midwife's waning patronage.[32]

Reformers failed to seek improvements among the different service providers, and did not work for centralized public administration to guarantee quality standards. Instead, as public health advocates searched for quality control, they all too readily embraced the medical expert. In order to achieve uniformity of care, certainly a valid goal in the early part of the century, they relied increasingly upon the hospital-affiliated physician and his assistants. Thus, while publicizing unnecessary deaths in childbirth, health officials told women not to become alarmed, but instead to see a doctor. "The doctor and nurse do for the woman what experts at the service station do for the automobile." Reformers' infatuation with expertise blinded them to midwives' possibilities as permanent grassroots health personnel. Ironically this ultimately undermined reformers' own hopes for equalizing access to health services and to quality health care.[33]

The public health movement proved effective in analyzing and publicizing the deficiencies of health care in America, and could claim credit for considerable health gains. Nevertheless, having bowed to medical experts without questioning their qualifications, public health activists abandoned to private medicine the improvements achieved in pilot demonstrations. More important, the public health movement never directly attacked the economic thesis that sustained the private physician: that high fees should be the reward for long and expensive training. Hence childbirth moved into the hospital, removed from public oversight, where the maturing obstetrical specialty could serve a paying clientele. All women suffered as a result of the unrestrained practice of the doctor, but poor women suffered especially. They became the clinical material for medical specialization, and lost birth attendants who were indigenous to their neighborhoods and cultures.[34]

Somehow the public health movement had to break the ubiquitous tradition of medical laissez-faire. By requiring public supervision of midwives, thus suggesting that health providers should be publicly accountable, health reformers might have furthered the cause. But the public health movement of the early twentieth century was too contradictory to do that. It bore the concept of health as human birthright, but failed to reconstruct organized medicine to serve the public interest. Succumbing to the medical expert in a private setting meant that health reform would later confine itself to seeking payment methods (voluntary insurance) for middle-class patients, increasingly priced out of expensive hospital care. Two systems of medical service resulted, catering to different social groups—one private, depending on one's ability to pay (at least for insurance), the other charitable, measured by the public budget, largess, and current politics. The public system, necessarily plagued with financial uncertainties and overworked and resentful staffs, could never offer its care generously. Burdened with administrative requirements that recipients qualify financially, public health never became more than a welfare gift.

To blame these conditions on a misogynous American medical system is tempting, yet facile. With support from the American Medical

Association, physicians concentrated on establishing medicine as an elite specialized discipline, free from government interference. Physicians' writings and especially their behavior—shown vividly in organized medical opposition to health insurance and even the relatively unthreatening Sheppard-Towner Act—showed lust for unrestricted power and status. Doctors inveighed against centralized supervision, while public health leaders relied readily on the premise (however erroneous) that childbirth in the hands of the expert, whose training and degree presumably conferred infallibility, meant safety. The doctors' victory doomed the midwife. She died because she posed a reasonable alternative to the physician, and because her existence necessarily required supervision—and outside review, once legitimated, might one day fall upon the doctor himself.

NOTES

1. For example, see Suzanne Arms, *Immaculate Deception: A New Look at Women and Childbirth in America* (Boston: Houghton Mifflin Co., 1975); Adrienne Rich, *Of Woman Born: Motherhood as Experience and Institution* (New York: W. W. Norton and Co., 1976); Sheila Kitzinger, *The Experience of Childbirth* (Middlesex, England: Pelican Books, 1977); Doris Haire, *The Cultural Warping of Childbirth* (Hillside, N.J.: International Childbirth Education Association, 1972); Gena Corea, *The Hidden Malpractice: How American Medicine Treats Women as Patients and Professionals* (New York: William Morrow and Co., 1977), pp. 184–219.

2. Leila J. Rupp supplies an appropriate definition of gender interpretation as one which emphasizes sex as "a primary category of analysis or explanatory factor for understanding the unequal and unjust distribution of power and resources in society. . . ." See "Reflections on Twentieth-Century American Women's History," *Reviews in American History* 9 (June 1981): 283. Historical interpretations that perceive explicitly misogynistic reasons for the destruction of the American midwife include Rich, *Of Woman Born*, pp. 136–41; G. J. Barker-Benfield, *The Horrors of the Half-Known Life: Male Attitudes Toward Women and Sexuality in Nineteenth-Century America* (New York: Harper & Row, 1976), pp. 61–71; and Barbara Ehrenreich and Deirdre English, *Witches, Midwives, and Nurses: A History of Women Healers* (Old Westbury, N.Y.: The Feminist Press, 1973), pp. 1–41. Although Ehrenreich and English see the campaign against the midwife as part of a larger class struggle aimed at grassroots and irregular healers, they contend that "when women healers were attacked, they were attacked as *women*" (p. 2). Again, they assert (p. 41): "Take away sexism and you take away one of the mainstays of the health hierarchy." Another example

is Ann Oakley, "Wisewoman and Medicine Man: Changes in the Management of Childbirth," in *The Rights and Wrongs of Women*, ed. Juliet Mitchell and Ann Oakley (Middlesex, England: Penguin Books, 1976), pp. 1–58. Jane B. Donegan, *Women and Men Midwives: Medicine, Morality, and Misogyny in Early America* (Westport, Conn.: Greenwood Press, 1978), adopts a more cautious approach to sexism in medicine. She believes that sexist definitions of women precluded midwives from the training that, with new scientific discoveries, they required to maintain the confidence of their clientele.

3.   Regina Morantz has done substantial work regarding women and medicine, and warns strenuously against misuse of psychological generalizations. Psychologizing often removes historical subjects from the concrete, from the social, cultural, political, and economic milieus, and may serve contemporary rather than historical investigations. See her essay questioning the validity of a psychological approach to the interpretation of medicine and women in the nineteenth century, "The Lady and Her Physician," in *Clio's Consciousness Raised: New Perspectives on the History of Women*, ed. Mary Hartman and Lois Banner (New York: Harper & Row, 1974), pp. 38–53. Again, one seeing male physicians guided by unconscious hostility toward women would expect women doctors to be different. Female physicians did not become midwives' defenders; moreover, their clinical practices did not differ substantially from those of their male counterparts. See Regina Markell Morantz and Sue Zschoche, "Professionalism, Feminism, and Gender Roles: A Comparative Study of Nineteenth-Century Medical Therapeutics," *Journal of American History* 67 (December 1980): 568–88. These authors find that women doctors have been guided by contemporary professional modes, not gender allegiance.

4.   For discussions of the new intellectual orientation produced by the understanding of bacteriological etiology, see Morris J. Vogel and Charles E. Rosenberg, eds., *The Therapeutic Revolution: Essays in the Social History of American Medicine* (Philadelphia: University of Pennsylvania Press, 1979). The following essays are particularly useful: Charles E. Rosenberg, "The Therapeutic Revolution: Medicine, Meaning, and Social Change in Nineteenth-Century America," pp. 3–25; Russell C. Maulitz, " 'Physician Versus Bacteriologist': The Ideology of Science in Clinical Medicine," pp. 91–107; and Edmund D. Pellegrino, "The Sociocultural Impact of Twentieth-Century Therapeutics," pp. 245–66.

5.   For secondary material discussing the development of the American medical profession, see James J. Walsh, *History of Medicine in New York: Three Centuries of Medical Progress*, 5 vols. (New York: National Americana Society, 1919); James G. Burrow, *AMA: Voice of American Medicine* (Baltimore: Johns Hopkins University Press, 1963); James G. Burrow, *Organized Medicine in the Progressive Era: The Move Toward Monopoly* (Baltimore: Johns Hopkins University Press, 1977); William G. Rothstein, *American Physicians in the Nineteenth Century: From Sects to Science*

(Baltimore: Johns Hopkins University Press, 1972); Martin Kaufman, *American Medical Education: The Formative Years, 1765–1910* (Westport, Conn.: Greenwood Press, 1976); Joseph F. Kett, *The Formation of the American Medical Profession: The Role of Institutions, 1780–1860* (New Haven: Yale University Press, 1968); John Duffy, *The Healers: The Rise of the Medical Establishment* (New York: McGraw-Hill, 1976).

6. For a discussion of the pivotal role of the AMA in medical "reform," see David K. Rosner and Gerald E. Markowitz, "Doctors in Crisis: A Study of the Use of Medical Education Reform to Establish Modern Professional Elitism in Medicine," *American Quarterly* 25 (March 1973): 83–107. Abraham Flexner, *Medical Education in the United States and Canada: A Report to the Carnegie Foundation for the Advancement of Teaching,* Bulletin No. 4 (New York: Carnegie Foundation, 1910).

7. Inez C. Philbrich, "A Municipally Salaried Obstetrical Staff," *Woman's Medical Journal* 26 (August 1916): 191; Arthur B. Emmons and James L. Huntington, "The Midwife, Her Future in the United States," *American Journal of Obstetrics and Diseases of Women and Children* 65 (March 1912): 394. By contrast the medical struggle against the British midwife came under the leadership of general practitioners who depended upon midwifery cases to bolster their precarious incomes. See Jean Donnison, *Midwives and Medical Men: A History of Inter-Professional Rivalries and Women's Rights* (New York: Schocken Books, 1977), pp. 116–17, 122.

8. John Van Doren Young, "The Midwife Problem in the State of New York," *New York State Journal of Medicine* 15 (August 1915): 291; Society of the Lying-In Hospital of the City of New York, *Annual Report for the Years 1922 and 1923,* p. 14. In 1922 Dr. J. Clifton Edgar, professor of obstetrics at Cornell University Medical School, also articulated this view: "Statistics are available to show that less than half of all pregnancies are normal." See introduction to Carolyn C. Van Blarcom, *Getting Ready to Be a Mother: A Little Book of Information and Advice for the Young Woman Who Is Looking Forward to Motherhood* (New York: MacMillan, 1922), p. xiv. Indeed, the first quarter of the twentieth century was the heyday of obstetrical operative interference (viz., resort to forceps, version, or Caesarean section). Analysis of maternal mortality in the late twenties identified the frequently unnecessary use of forceps and Caesarean section as major causes. Denigrations of midwives' capabilities appear in Emmons and Huntington, "The Midwife, Her Future," p. 394, and Thomas Darlington, "The Present Status of the Midwife," *American Journal of Obstetrics and Diseases of Women and Children* 58 (May 1911): 873.

9. J. Milton Mabbott, "The Regulation of Midwives in New York," *American Journal of Obstetrics and Diseases of Women and Children* 55 (April 1907): 526–27. See also Young, "The Midwife Problem," p. 294; Ralph W. Lobenstine, "The Influence of the Midwife upon Infant and Maternal Morbidity and Mortality," *American Journal of Obstetrics and*

Diseases of Women and Children 58 (October 1911): 878; Henry J. Garrigues, *A Text-Book of the Science and Art of Obstetrics* (Philadelphia: J. B. Lippincott Co., 1902), p. 214.

10. E. R. Hardin, "The Midwife Problem," *Southern Medical Journal* 18 (May 1925): 349. The assumption that midwives deprived women of the best that science could offer is expressed in Mabbott, "The Regulation of Midwives in New York," pp. 526–27: "The writer of this paper believes that a woman should be examined during pregnancy and that urinalysis should be made in every case. I believe that a woman in confinement is entitled to professional care. I believe she is entitled to some relief of suffering . . . including the use of chloroform. . . . Still further, I believe that immediate [surgery] should be done in . . . cases of laceration of the perineum which cannot be predicted in advance. How can I, therefore, recommend a law for the license and regulation of midwives when they regularly deprive women of some or all of these advantages?"

11. Hardin, "The Midwife Problem," p. 347; Emmons and Huntington, "The Midwife, Her Future," p. 396.

12. Joseph B. DeLee, "Progress Toward Ideal Obstetrics," *American Journal of Obstetrics and Diseases of Women and Children* 73 (March 1916): 410; J. L. Huntington, "The Midwife in Massachusetts: Her Anomalous Position," *Boston Medical and Surgical Journal* 168 (March 20, 1913): 419.

13. Charles E. Ziegler, "How We Can Best Solve the Midwifery Problem," *American Journal of Public Health* 12 (May 1922): 407, 409; see also Mabbott, "The Regulation of Midwives in New York," pp. 526–27; Hardin, "The Midwife Problem," p. 348; Young, "The Midwife Problem," p. 294.

14. For discussions of the prevalence of midwifery practice in immigrant communities, see P. R. Eastman, *A Comparison of the Birth Rates of Native and Foreign-Born White Women in the State of New York During 1916* (Albany: Department of Health, 1916), p. 4: Native white women total births (excluding New York City), 64,888; by midwife, 2,504, or 3.9 percent. Foreign-born women total births, 37,194; by midwife, 14,165, or 37.3 percent; East Harlem Nursing and Health Demonstration, *The Maternity Service Report of the East Harlem Nursing and Health Demonstration* (New York: The East Harlem Nursing and Health Demonstration, 1928); Michael Davis, *Immigrant Health and the Community* (New York: Harper and Brothers, 1921; reprint ed., Montclair, N.J.: Paterson Smith Publishing Co., 1971); Grace Abbott, "The Midwife in Chicago," *American Journal of Sociology* 20 (March 1915): 684.

15. U.S. Department of Labor, Children's Bureau, *Standards of Child Welfare, A Report of the Children's Bureau Conference, May and June, 1919, Section III, "The Control of Midwifery,"* by Henry D. Chapin, Publication No. 220 (Washington, D.C.: Government Printing Office, 1919);

also S. Josephine Baker, "Schools for Midwives," *American Journal of Obstetrics and Diseases of Women and Children* 65 (February 1912): 257.

16.   See U.S. Department of Labor, Children's Bureau, *Infant-Welfare Work in Europe: An Account of Recent Experiences in Great Britain, Austria, Belgium, France, Germany, and Italy*, by Nettie McGill, Publication No. 76 (Washington, D.C.: Government Printing Office, 1921), for descriptions of requirements for midwives in various foreign countries; also Children's Bureau, *Standards of Child Welfare*, Discussion, Arthur Newsholme in response to Chapin, p. 164. In 1902, when Parliament passed the Midwives Act and created a Central Midwives Board, the English midwife gained official status. In 1919 the maternal mortality per 1,000 live births stood at 4.4 in England and Wales against 7.4 in the United States birth registration area (which incorporated the most developed and wealthiest regions of the country). See Elizabeth Hunt, *Public Maternity and Infant Care in Berlin and Stockholm* (New York: American-Scandinavian Foundation, 1922), p. 6.

17.   Midwifery legislation in New York City represented the most thorough American attempt at legitimation. By an act of June 6, 1907, the New York Legislature defined the midwife as one assisting in normal childbirth and receiving compensation. The statute banned the midwife's use of forceps or any mechanical device, as well as any drug but disinfectants, and restricted her to simple delivery situations. The law gave special authority to the New York City Department of Health to establish its own rules governing midwives. The following year, the City Health Department acted. The city regulations limited practice to holders of Board of Health permits, valid for only one year. Before licensing, the midwife worked under a physician, with clinical observation of at least twenty cases of labor and twenty ten-day follow-ups of mothers and infants. The rules narrowed midwives' attendance to cases of normal vertex (head) presentations. After 1911, when Bellevue Hospital opened the first public school of midwifery, New York City required that midwife applicants have been graduated from Bellevue or a comparable European school. See An Act Regulating and Restraining the Practice of Midwifery in the City of New York, L. 1907, ch. 432, and *Rules and Regulations Governing the Practice of Midwifery in the City of New York, Adopted by the Board of Health* (New York: Department of Health, 1908), pp. 3–6, 9–13; John A. Foote, "Legislative Measures Against Maternal and Infant Mortality: The Midwife Practice Laws in the States and Territories of the United States," *American Journal of Obstetrics and Diseases of Women and Children* 80 (November 1919): 543–44, 546–48. In the south significant work with midwives began only after the tide had turned against the urban midwife. Southern midwives served rural populations too dispersed and poor to support the private physician. Work with the southern midwife after the passage of Sheppard-Towner lay outside the midwife debate, since southern midwives, even when trained, posed little threat to the medical

profession. For descriptions of the work with southern midwives under Sheppard-Towner, see a series of articles published in the *Medical Woman's Journal* 33 and 34 (1926–27).

18. J. M. Baldy, "Is the Midwife a Necessity?" *American Journal of Obstetrics and Diseases of Women and Children* 73 (March 1916): 406; Linsly R. Williams, "The Position of the New York State Department of Health Relative to the Control of Midwives," *New York State Journal of Medicine* 14 (August 1915): 298.

19. J. Clifton Edgar, "The Education, Licensing and Supervision of the Midwife," *American Journal of Obstetrics and Diseases of Women and Children* 78 (March 1916): 386–88, 395–96, 398; also Baldy, "Is the Midwife a Necessity?" pp. 400, 406.

20. The present approach views health reformers as part of the progressive thrust to deal with an impersonal society created by urban and industrial conditions; health reform became part of the "search for order," led by "disinterested" experts. See Robert H. Wiebe, *The Search for Order, 1877–1920* (New York: Hill and Wang, 1967).

21. *Seventh Annual Report of the New York Milk Committee for the Year Ending December 31, 1913*, p. 42. The Maternity Center Association, founded in New York City in 1918 and incorporated in 1919, pleaded with women to visit maternity centers for prenatal care even if they planned to use midwives. The centers in turn employed female physicians to make immigrant patients more comfortable and to acclimate them to the notion of physicians attending childbirth. See Maternity Center Association, *A Fair Chance for Your Baby and You: Twelve Helpful Talks* (New York: Maternity Center Association, 1922), p. 2.

22. E. H. Lewinski-Corwin, *The Hospital Situation in Greater New York: Report of a Survey of Hospitals in New York City by the Public Health Committee of the New York Academy of Medicine* (New York: G. P. Putnam's Sons, 1924), p. 64; Children's Bureau, *Standards of Child Welfare*, S. Josephine Baker, p. 165: "By the constant supervision of the midwife, and the elimination from practice of every midwife who violates our regulations, the number of practicing midwives has been reduced in ten years from 3,000 to 1,600."

23. Discussion, S. Josephine Baker, in Mrs. Max West, "The Development of Prenatal Care in the United States," *American Association for the Study and Prevention of Infant Mortality, Transactions of the Fifth Annual Meeting, Boston, Mass., November 12–14, 1914*, p. 113. Jacob Sobel, *Instruction and Supervision of Expectant Mothers in New York City* (New York: Department of Health, Monograph Series No. 21, 1919), pp. 17–18. (The study does not account for the remaining 9 percent.) The rate of puerperal sepsis per 10,000 births, by attendant: midwives, 1915, 8.6; 1916, 10.7; doctors, 1915, 24.0; 1916, 20.6.

24. See Davis, *Immigrant Health and the Community*, pp. 205, 213;

Williams, "The Position of the N. Y. State Department of Health Relative to the Control of Midwives," p. 300; Julius Levy, "The Maternal and Infant Mortality in Midwifery Practice in Newark, New Jersey," *American Journal of Obstetrics and Diseases of Women and Children* 77 (January 1918): 41–42.

25. Carolyn C. Van Blarcom, "A Possible Solution to the Midwife Problem," *Proceedings of the National Conference of Charities and Correction at the 37th Annual Session, St. Louis, Mo., May 19–26, 1919*, p. 350. Van Blarcom served as executive secretary of the Committee on the Prevention of Blindness of the New York Association for the Blind. Davis, *Immigrant Health*, p. 214; "Conservation of Eyesight," *Survey* 25 (Feb. 7, 1911): 522; "Infant Blindness in Massachusetts," *Survey* 25 (Oct. 1, 1910): 9, quote from Sobel, *Instruction and Supervision*, p. 18.

26. William Allen Pusey, "Some of the Social Problems of Medicine," *Journal of the American Medical Association* (hereafter *JAMA*) (June 14, 1924): 1906. For an excellent analysis of organized medicine's ambivalence toward public health reform, see John Duffy, "The American Medical Profession and Public Health: From Support to Ambivalence," *Bulletin of the History of Medicine* 53 (Spring 1979): 1–22. For the medical profession's response to proposed schemes of health insurance, see Ronald L. Numbers, *Almost Persuaded: American Physicians and Compulsory Health Insurance, 1912–1920* (Baltimore: Johns Hopkins University Press, 1978). For a full description of the Sheppard-Towner Act, see *Text of the Act for the Promotion of the Welfare and Hygiene of Maternity and Infancy. And of Supplementary Legislation*, U.S. Department of Labor, Children's Bureau, *The Promotion of the Welfare and Hygiene of Maternity and Infancy: The Administration of the Act of Congress of November 23, 1921, for the Fiscal Year Ended June 30, 1926*, Publication No. 178 (Washington, D.C.: Government Printing Office, 1927), pp. 85–87.

27. Kosmak, who died at eighty-one on July 10, 1954, served as editor of the *American Journal of Obstetrics and Diseases of Women and Children* from 1909 until its discontinuance in 1919. In 1920 he founded the *American Journal of Obstetrics and Gynecology* and edited it until 1952. He also edited the *New York State Journal of Medicine* from 1945 until 1952 and the *Bulletin of the Lying-In Hospital* from 1904 to 1932. See Manuscript Collection, New York Academy of Medicine, Box 8, New York Obstetrical Society Folder, "In Memoriams," 1924–54. Letter to the editor, George W. Kosmak, "The Sheppard-Towner Bill," *JAMA* 76 (May 7, 1921): 1319; letter to the editor, George W. Kosmak, "Sheppard-Towner Bill," *New York Times* (August 5, 1921).

28. U.S. Congress, House, *Hearings Before the Committee on Interstate and Foreign Commerce*, 67th Cong., 1st Sess., 1921, statement of George W. Kosmak, p. 100.

29. These articles demonstrate the tenor of AMA reaction to the

Sheppard-Towner Act: Editorial, "The Sheppard-Towner Bill," *JAMA* 76 (May 28, 1921): 1504; "Four Million Women to Push Maternity Act," *JAMA* 87 (Oct. 30, 1926): 1488; editorial, "The Perpetuation of the Sheppard-Towner Idea," *JAMA* 87 (Nov. 27, 1926): 1833; editorial, "Protest the Sheppard-Towner Act," *JAMA* 89 (Feb. 6, 1926): 421; editorial, "Again, Protest the Sheppard-Towner Act," *JAMA* 86 (May 8, 1926): 1458; "Sheppard-Towner Bill Side-tracked," *JAMA* 87 (July 3, 1926): 41; "Women's Clubs Urge Extension of the Sheppard-Towner Act," *JAMA* 87 (Dec. 11, 1926): 2008. While Sheppard-Towner was by its terms permanent, the statute provided that funding after June 30, 1927, would depend upon congressional decision. Proponents decided to move for renewal authorization a year earlier, in 1926. After heated debate legislators compromised on a two-year extension, which carried an automatic repealer effective June 30, 1929.

30. Clara D. Noyes served as general superintendent of Training Schools for Bellevue and Allied Hospitals in New York City; Van Blarcom, besides her role in preventing unnecessary infant blindness, was also assistant secretary of the Section on Midwifery of the American Association for the Study and Prevention of Infant Mortality; Grace Abbott made a career of infant-welfare work, and upon the retirement of Julia Lathrop as head of the United States Children's Bureau assumed the post; Baker headed the New York City Bureau of Child Hygiene, and Sobel was a division chief; Levy served as the first director of Newark's Bureau of Child Hygiene. While Donnison makes clear that the British Midwives' Act of 1902 was less of a victory for midwifery than commonly depicted by American admirers, she shows that British midwives might have succumbed to the same fate as their American counterparts had it not been for the well-organized efforts of defenders (particularly middle-class women) outside their ranks. See *Midwives and Medical Men*, pp. 40–41, 87, 174–75, 177–79.

31. For unequivocal defenses of midwives' capacities, see Mary Breckinridge, "The Nurse-Midwife—A Pioneer," *American Journal of Public Health* 17 (November 1927): 1149; Mary Breckinridge, *Wide Neighborhoods: A Story of the Frontier Nursing Service* (New York: Harper and Brothers, 1952); and Mary Beard, *The Nurse in Public Health* (New York: Harper and Brothers, 1929), pp. 113, 116, 133, 136, 162. In her valuable study of American midwives, Judy Barrett Litoff finds genuine division over midwives among public health officials. Litoff contends that while some health leaders argued for midwife regulation only until medical replacement, others, employing low-mortality, midwife-dominated European countries as models, urged full training and incorporation of the midwife into the American medical scene. See *American Midwives, 1860 to the Present* (Westport, Conn.: Greenwood Press, 1978). The present author's research, however, suggests that this group, a distinct minority, failed to organize successfully to promote its cause. For an earlier study depicting the factions in the midwife

debate, see Frances E. Kobrin, "The American Midwife Controversy: A Crisis of Professionalization," *Bulletin of the History of Medicine* 40 (July–August 1966): 350–63.

32. S. Josephine Baker, *Fighting for Life* (New York: Macmillan, 1929), pp. 112–13.

33. Maternity Center Association, A *Fair Chance for Your Baby and You*, p. 2. This blind recommendation may not have been so harmful if the expert practiced in the public sphere, outside the grip of private medicine. But the expert to whom health reformers began to defer lay in the private sector of medicine, so health reform would benefit primarily a wealthy clientele.

34. The public health movement proved most effective in lowering death rates from contagious diseases in the first year of life. Between 1890 and 1913, the death rate fell from 46.3 to 17.9 per 100,000 population for typhoid fever; for diphtheria and croup from 97.8 to 18.8; for tuberculosis from 252 to 147.6; and for pneumonia from 186.9 to 132.4. In the birth registration area of the United States, infant mortality fell from 100 per 1,000 live births in 1915 to 65 in 1927. In New York City, where perhaps the most intensive public health work occurred, infant mortality fell from 144 in 1908 to 110 in 1912, 98.2 in 1914, 94.6 in 1915, 93.1 in 1916, 88.8 in 1917, 91.7 in 1918, and 81.6 in 1919. See Ernst Christopher Meyer, *Infant Mortality in New York City: A Study of Results Accomplished by Infant-Life Saving Agencies, 1885–1920* (New York: Rockefeller Foundation, Publication No. 10, 1921).

5

False Dawn: The Rise and Decline of Public Health Nursing in America, 1900–1930

Karen Buhler-Wilkerson

In "the long view of history, the grey clad nurse with the cross on her arm—climbing the stairs of the city tenement . . . may perhaps prove the symbolic figure of the century in which the results of a new science of healing were applied in a new and universal fashion to promote the well-being of mankind." This is how C.-E. A. Winslow, an eminent public health leader, thought the nurses of his time would be remembered. In retrospect his optimistic picture appears to have been little more than wishful thinking.[1]

Yet, at the turn of the century, the future did hold great promise for public health nursing. To the public and the voluntary agencies who sought their services, these nurses seemed to be an economical and appropriate way to help the poor. While caring for the sick, the nurse could teach the family rules of personal hygiene, thus protecting both healthy family members and the public at large from the spread of infectious disease. Within a decade the public health nurse's role had expanded to include a variety of preventive services, not only for those suffering from infectious diseases like tuberculosis, but also for mothers, babies, schoolchildren, and industrial workers. Since public health nurses fit neatly into the system of social and medical care that was evolving at the time, it was not surprising that the number and variety of agencies seeking their services increased steadily.[2]

By the late 1920s, however, public health nursing had reached a turning point. It was becoming apparent that a movement that might have been significant in delivering comprehensive health care to the

American public would fail to reach its potential. With the end of immigration, the growing importance of the hospital, and the declining significance of infectious disease, public health nurses found their work relegated to an increasingly marginal role in the health care system. Hence, this paper will examine some of the factors that shaped both the rise and decline of public health nursing between 1900–1930.[3]

I

Agencies to provide nursing care for the poor were first organized in the United States in the late nineteenth century. Located in northeastern urban areas, where the concentration of immigrants and industry made poverty, disease, and dirt unavoidable, visiting or district nursing associations began as small undertakings in which a few wealthy women would hire one or two nurses to visit the sick poor in their homes. In most associations the nurses worked six to six and a half days a week, eight to ten hours a day, and were able to visit eight to twelve patients each day. The ailments they encountered were frequently infectious, often acute, and always complicated by the social and economic circumstances of the family.[4]

For a variety of reasons the complex nursing problems presented by the poverty-stricken patients these associations served were thought to require skill and experience beyond that of the average trained nurse. For one thing, visiting nurses, unlike private duty nurses, rarely had a doctor at hand or even the "appliances" of the hospital or the middle-class private home. For another, visiting nurses were supposed to do more than care for the indigent sick. As was the case with so many philanthropic activities, the visiting nurse was meant to bring a message with her medicines. A disciplined and well-bred woman, she was expected to raise the "household existence" with her delicate instruction and firm conviction, and to protect the public from the spread of disease with her forceful yet tactful lessons in physical and moral hygiene. A story frequently used in agency fund-raising material described a woman who worked in a candy store, boarded with friends, and was found by the nurse to have tuberculosis. The need for visiting nurses was dramatized by the accompanying warning: "think of all the tuberculosis bacilli presented with each package of candy."[5]

Of course, with the cost of hospital care rising at this time, the visiting nurse was also seen as an economical solution to the medical needs of urban workers. Prior to the turn of the century, voluntary hospitals had been primarily charitable institutions. But as hospitals faced increasingly severe "deficit problems," they became less tolerant of patients who could not pay for their care. Some contemporary spokesmen even asserted that hospitals were in economic trouble because they had been involved in too much charity work. Obviously, therefore, one way to relieve hospital burdens was to provide the poor with more care in their own homes, while simultaneously teaching them how to stay healthy.[6]

As knowledge of their work spread, visiting nurses became popular figures. Mary Gardner, director of the Providence Visiting Nurse Association, recalled that during the first decade of the twentieth century, "support . . . became easy." According to Gardner, "all sorts of groups not previously concerned with nursing or indeed health or sickness in any form, engaged a nurse and sent her forth to produce whatever result she was capable of producing." In 1909 Lillian Wald, founder of the Henry Street Settlement, even convinced the Metropolitan Life Insurance Company to provide the service of trained nurses as an additional benefit to its industrial policyholders. The mutual advantages of the arrangements were readily apparent. At a cost of five cents a policy, the Metropolitan could reduce the number of death benefits it had to pay. And without additional fund-raising efforts, district nursing associations could extend services to more of the working population. By 1911, "Mother Met," as the company was affectionately called, had decided to offer its nursing services throughout the entire country. Where possible it arranged for existing visiting nursing associations to provide the care; where that was not possible, it hired its own nurses. Three years after the service was initiated, the Metropolitan was paying for one million nursing visits each year at a cost of roughly $500,000 per year.[7]

Thus, with many social, economic and medical factors encouraging a growing demand for public health nurses during the first decade of the twentieth century, the number of agencies hiring public health nurses increased from only fifty-eight in 1901 to nearly two thousand by 1914. Public health nurses could be found working for department stores, industries, insurance companies, boards of health and education, hospitals, settlement houses, milk and baby committees, playgrounds, and hotels, as well as visiting nurse associations. In fact there were sixty different associations employing public health nurses in New York City alone.[8]

This rapid, even hectic and confusing growth brought more services to the poor, and it led to the development of an important new field of employment for nurses. But it also created what would become an increasingly severe problem. Evolving agency by agency, public health nursing grew up outside the control of the nursing profession. To be sure, visiting nurses were given increasing responsibility for the management of patient care. As Mary Beard, director of Boston's Instructive District Nurse Association, suggested, they were becoming "a really dynamic force." Nevertheless, if the women philanthropists who managed visiting nurse agencies no longer expected to "oversee" the daily practice of "their nurses," they did maintain control of agency administration. With lay women hiring, firing, financing, and setting agency policy, nurses had no way of determining the future development of these agencies or of visiting nursing as a field. Moreover, although leading visiting nurses saw real danger in this situation, they did not act early enough or in sufficiently organized fashion to influence development in a truly significant way.[9]

The vulnerable situation of visiting nursing began to be seriously discussed by nurses in 1911. As one member of the board of the Cleveland Visiting Nurse Association observed at the time: "We find quite suddenly that matters of method and of ethics can be left to the mercy of general interpretation only so long as no powerful suggestion to construe them unusually is made from without." Her rather vague words of warning were, in fact, a response to just such a suggestion. Ella Crandall and Lillian Wald, both leading public health nurses, had recently learned of a proposal made by Dr. Lee Frankel, vice president of the Metropolitan Life Insurance Company, to the boards of the Chicago and Boston visiting nurse associations. Addressing his request to two associations that were in the midst of reorganization and without the guidance of a superintendent of nurses, Frankel had asked the boards to add practical nurses to their staffs to take care of chronic patients. By thus hiring less expensive attendants, Frankel hoped to reduce the cost of the nursing services that the Metropolitan had agreed to provide to its industrial policyholders during illness. The nursing profession could no longer ignore the influence of "Mother Met."[10]

Responding swiftly to Frankel's plan, leaders of organized nursing discussed the matter privately with Frankel and publicly in nursing journals. For example, Edna Foley, the superintendent-elect of the Chicago association, wrote an article in which the proposal's risks to patients were made clear. Foley rhetorically queried whether Frankel's request meant that visiting nurse associations were "intended to care for the sick or to act as investigating agents and supervisors for commercial interest?" And she then asked whether standards had been "so lowered that only the number of visits and the amount of instruction given counts, while the actual work of our hands has become so unimportant that it can with safety and expedition be handed over to so-called practical nurses, whose practice is on a par with the scanty remuneration they receive?" In conclusion she asserted: "the poor are at the mercy of too many half-trained and counterfeit workers as it is, and it behooves the visiting nurse associations in good standing to maintain the integrity of our calling by offering their best alike to the acute and the chronic sick."[11]

Despite their strong stand against the Metropolitan proposal, nurses did recognize that many chronic patients could get along without expensive expert care. Nevertheless, since they were still struggling to convince the public that expert nursing care was important, nurses felt called upon to resist this potential threat to fragile public confidence. At a New York Academy of Medicine meeting, Annie Goodrich, a leading nurse, described their position this way:

> If there is another body or class of workers needed, it will come into existence; we believe, indeed, that such a class is here and is only waiting to come into an orderly existence for the field of the more important worker, the nurse, to be developed. . . . If the doctor and the family are satisfied to relegate their sick into her hands, well and good. Our responsibility ceases. Our point has been made when the line of demarcation is clear.

Obviously no such line of demarcation as the one Goodrich called for had been made for public health nurses. Indeed, Frankel's efforts to develop a special kind of nursing care for the chronically ill pushed to the forefront an issue of professional self-definition that visiting nurses were not yet prepared to resolve.[12]

In the end Frankel was convinced to drop his plan, although he did succeed in reducing the company's expenditures for the care of chronic patients. Arguing that services to the acutely ill demonstrated larger practical returns, services to the chronically ill were virtually eliminated. More importantly, however, Frankel's proposal provided the impetus needed to convince visiting nurses to organize themselves. As Isabel Lowman described what many had learned, organization was now thought necessary if "the treasures of their tradition" were to "be preserved intact."[13]

In January 1912, Lillian Wald became chairwoman of a committee formed by the American Nurses' Association and the American Society of Superintendents of Training Schools for nurses to consider the possibility of cooperation, and by June the National Organization for Public Health Nursing had been created. The organization's name had been hotly debated. Tradition and sentiment argued for the term "visiting nurse," but that term was eventually dropped in favor of one thought big enough to cover all the work being done. As Ella Crandall explained it, in the term finally chosen to describe the new organization the nurses were "borrowing from or banking on the future, rather than the past or present [and] . . . establishing in anticipation a vital connection between visiting nursing and public health."[14]

II

It was the changing emphasis of the "public health campaign" that created the possibility of this new bond between visiting nurses and public health. As the focus of the public health movement shifted from what C.-E. A. Winslow had once graphically described as "the swamp and the dung heap" to the "hygienic guidance of the individual living machine," it had come to require a new worker, a teacher of prevention. The visiting nurse seemed a logical choice for this new role. But, health nursing, as Winslow liked to call it, differed so greatly from sick nursing that it might one day constitute a distinct profession. Indeed the nurse entering this new field was establishing a unique area of practice, one in which her increased autonomy from the medical profession was expected to distinguish her work from other kinds of public health activity. The public health nurse's special role would be to teach individuals how to reduce their susceptibility to disease through alterations in daily habits. Promoting good personal hygiene, fresh air, sunshine, cleanliness, exercise, and proper diet would be the focus of the nurse's work. As one medical authority suggested, public health nurses would serve as "the relay station, to carry the power from the central stations of science, the hospitals, and the universities to the individual homes of the community."[15]

In actuality, though, nurses who specialized in this new preventive role found it difficult to combine educative functions with care for the "bodily needs" of patients. To many it seemed unreasonable to think that nurses would really take time for health teaching while their sick patients were waiting for a bath or treatment, and increasingly the roles diverged. Some leading public health nurses warned against this separation, declaring that divorcing instructive work from bedside nursing was a great mistake. They were warned that the best public health nurses might become scientists or teachers at the expense of more traditional delivery functions, thus allowing their profession to fall victim to the specialization they saw as a characteristic peril of the age.[16]

But health officers, at least some of them, favored specialization. They argued that nurses who spent any significant part of their time providing bedside care should not be classified as public health nurses. Such a role was therapeutic rather than hygienic and dealt with individuals rather than the maintenance of health in the well population. Concomitantly, the Americanization movement provided added legitimization for the new nursing role, in which teaching was the primary interest. As the agent of Americanization, it was argued, a visiting nurse could teach the immigrants self-help and health skills in terms of life's daily routines. Michael Davis, director of the Boston Dispensary, would later even go so far as to declare that the employment of visiting nurses was the "most important single step made by health departments toward effective methods of work with the immigrant."[17]

With much to support a growing demand for nurses whose primary focus was prevention, new training programs began to be called for, since few programs included any experiences of this type. Although it was unclear what training for public health work should ideally include, it was clear that it should involve more than training in the bedside care of the hospitalized sick. By 1912, several of the larger visiting nursing associations had initiated postgraduate courses in public health, but few training schools offered experience relevant to this new role. Hence most public health nurses continued to learn as they worked.[18]

For employers who hired large numbers of visiting nurses, this lack of job preparedness could result in considerable expense. As Elizabeth Crowell pointed out at a 1912 nursing convention, the New York Health Department "has had to conduct the actual training of 350 nurses employed by it because it felt that they were lacking in some respects." According to Crowell, that should not be. For the next five years, health departments, visiting nurse associations, and nursing organizations tried to improve this situation, but with little success, and United States entrance into World War I intensified the problems.[19]

III

The magnified demand for public health workers that was created by the war spawned a variety of plans for training non-nurse health workers. One such plan, which was supported most actively by Haven

Emerson, commissioner of health for New York City, involved the use of a new type of non-nurse worker, who would be trained to do the preventive and educational portion of public health visiting. Under this plan only the bedside care of the sick would remain under the aegis of public health nurses.[20]

Emerson discussed his proposal with Adelaide Nutting in July 1917, and by the end of the month Nutting, in turn, had shared the proposal with nurses across the country. Although sympathetic with the emergency situation that had precipitated Emerson's action, the nurses who responded found his solution unacceptable. On August 1, 1917, Emerson wrote Nutting expressing appreciation for her painstaking inquiry and her suggestions for an alternative course. The foregoing notwithstanding, Emerson told Nutting that he had decided to go ahead,

> to try, in a modest way, . . . a course for the preparation of public health workers, based upon higher educational requirements than those usually demanded by the nurses' training schools, the course to take two years and be planned along radically different lines from those at present followed, or likely to be followed, while nurses are prepared under the auspices of training schools.

Graduates would work under the supervision of nurses or doctors, and since according to Emerson they probably would not remain very long in service, their salary would consequently be small, $700 to $750. Thus Emerson hoped to provide in half the time, and at a significant savings, a worker who would be prepared to meet the health department's exact specifications.[21]

Because he was removed from office when a Tammany administration returned in January 1918, Emerson was unable to implement his plan. But he was not alone in his interest in developing non-nurse public health workers. Courses for college graduates similar to the one Emerson had proposed were being suggested in Wisconsin, California, and Virginia; and in France the Rockefeller Foundation's Committee for Tuberculosis and the American Red Cross Children's Bureau were establishing a ten-month course for health visitors.[22]

At roughly the same time, Dr. John Dill Robertson, another physician who was commissioner of health in Chicago, came up with what he thought was an even better idea. Believing, as did many physicians, that any bright, competent woman could be trained for nursing in a few months, Robertson decided to take advantage of what he called the "auspicious times" to establish a new school. It was called the Chicago

Training School for Home and Public Health Nursing and claimed to be able to produce a capable nurse in two months—4,231 of them in the first year. Trained nurses feared Robertson's panacea would hurt the profession and later found great delight in telling the story of a woman who called up one of the Chicago hospitals and said she had illness in her family and wanted a good nurse, adding, "Don't send me one of them public health nurses, as I am one myself."[23]

But in 1918, Robertson's proposal, combined with Emerson's plan and other developments actually underway, led many public health nurses to become alarmed. A nurse from Virginia expressed their concern with unusual clarity when she said:

> . . . in other words, the college women were to take over the highest functions of the nurse, those of teacher and leader, after a brief "course" as though these highest functions were so little technical that they might be laid in a few months as a durable veneer upon the foundation of a college education. This idea expanded would strip from the nursing profession the field of public health and lower the dignity of the bedside care of the sick.

Even George Vincent of the Rockefeller Foundation, who approached the problem from a different perspective, believed that unless the nursing profession found a suitable way to prepare public health nurses in large numbers they were certain to be replaced by non-nurse health visitors.[24]

Opposed to the idea of a health visitor without formal nursing training, organized nursing was willing to compromise. If a partially trained woman was needed, it was argued, her place should be at the bedside of convalescent and chronic patients, where she could be supervised by a highly trained nurse. The creation of an assistant, whose activities nursing could potentially control through licensure, training, and supervision, was far less threatening than the continued growth of a new competitive profession.[25]

Hence in 1918 the National Organization for Public Health Nursing reluctantly issued a statement accepting the employment of such attendants and establishing rules for their work in public health agencies. Soon thereafter, especially during the 1918 epidemic, visiting nurse associations began to hire untrained or partially trained workers. Probably the largest such undertaking was the supervised attendant service initiated by the Cleveland Visiting Nurse Association, with a registry of forty-six women.[26]

IV

The end of the First World War did not mark the end of the issues ignited by it. Having once allowed a differentiation among nursing functions, curative services being separated from preventive and acute from chronic, a situation had been created in which the role of the public health nurse could be divided into its component parts, and these then transferred to less educated and less expensive workers. If wartime plans to use non-nurse workers were continued in peacetime, the once multifaceted role of the public health nurse would be severely constricted.

In December 1918, therefore, the Rockefeller Foundation called a meeting to address some of the issues facing public health nurses. The foundation was interested in the matter because nurses provided a vital ancillary service in the public health programs it supported. It believed that with little agreement among those most interested in nursing's development, a conference might serve as a first step toward the kind of consensus that would result in an improved and unitary paradigm for public health nursing training. As anticipated the meeting dealt with a number of questions of interest to the foundation, but no consensus could be reached. Consequently a committee was appointed to study the questions the meeting had raised. Its final report was written by Josephine Goldmark and became widely known as the Goldmark Report.[27]

The study produced no real surprises, but it did, as one reviewer noted, reaffirm what nursing leaders had been saying for years. The committee recommended "that the teacher of hygiene in the home should possess, in the first place, the fundamental education of the nurse" supplemented by a graduate course in the special problems of public health. And it recommended, in addition, that a subsidiary worker should be used by public health agencies to assist the nurse with cases of mild and chronic illness. By the time the study was completed, however, these issues had become irrelevant. The once pressing need for either a health visitor or an attendant no longer existed. By 1922, the supply of public health nurses had significantly increased and their salaries were so low that it would have been difficult to introduce a new position that paid much less. As long as the labor supply remained high and the salary low, public health work would clearly remain the trained nurse's domain.[28]

By the end of the 1920s, a consensus seemed to be forming not only as to who the public health nurse should be but also as to what she should do. This consensus prescribed a role in which preventive care was emphasized, although bedside care was not ruled out. The diminished significance assigned to the bedside care of the sick did not arise from an abandonment of a desire to be the "community mother, the trained and scientific representative of the good neighbor" C.-E. A. Winslow had once described. It arose, rather, from the inability of organized nursing to create an institutional framework that would have allowed nurses to give equal attention to preventive and curative work. By the end of the decade, it was obvious that a dual-function public health nursing role would remain more a universal nursing ideal than an obtainable reality.[29]

In part, of course, nurses could gain few allies in their efforts to develop such agencies. The social, medical, and demographic circumstances that had created a need for large numbers of "community mothers" twenty years earlier were simply no longer of major concern to most communities. Urban death rates were dramatically declining and infectious diseases were being replaced by chronic degenerative diseases as the leading causes of death. These noninfectious diseases did not have the same kind of fluctuating, dramatic, and often frightening impact that had originally helped to prompt public concern and philanthropic support for the work of the visiting nurse. World War I and the immigration quota initiated in 1921 and 1924 also contributed to the changing nature of public health nursing. Fewer new immigrants and second-generation families meant the needs of the foreign-born could no longer help to legitimate the role of the nurse as the agent of Americanization. Finally, the hospital had also undergone a major transformation since the turn of the century. An institution that once housed the destitute sick poor was becoming a center of research and of clinical application for ideas and inventions derived from science and medical technology. What is more, by the 1930s, the number of hospital beds was growing six times faster than the population, and medical, surgical, and even some obstetrical patients, of all classes, were seeking hospital-based care. In the future fewer patients sick at home would require the skilled services of a trained nurse.[30]

Although their absolute numbers continued to increase, the logarithmical demand for public health nurses had peaked. By the 1920s, the proportion of public health nurses to the population had stabilized at an average of one nurse for every ten thousand people. Equally important, the work of many voluntary nursing agencies was no longer expanding. Their once clear purpose and vision had become increasingly elusive and financial support was becoming difficult to obtain. In some communities a new method of securing support was introduced through cooperative fund raising and the formation of community chests. In others, some voluntary agencies began to charge patients for nursing care. Called hourly services, the latter solution to dwindling income might increase an agency's revenue, but it also put the "visiting nurse" in competition with the private duty nurse for the increasingly small pool of paying patients who were sick at home.[31]

None of these approaches was very successful and even before the depression accelerated the trend, some visiting nurse associations began to shift their preventive services to government health departments. Not surprisingly, therefore, a survey of public health nursing conducted in 1931 found that the services of voluntary agencies were indeed becoming predominantly those having to do with the care of the sick. Although agencies claimed that the care for sick included family instruction in prevention, the investigators concluded that most "visiting nurses" did little teaching. Obviously such findings suggested the declining importance of the voluntary agencies and made it increasingly difficult to claim that "visiting nurses" were really public health nurses.[32]

While the number of new privately funded agencies declined, the number of local and state boards of health and education employing public health nurses increased. Predominantly involved with the delivery of preventive services, these public agencies were becoming the major arena for public health nurses' practice. In publicly funded jobs, public health nurses could find support for their traditional concerns—infectious diseases and health education for the poor. Even with such jobs open to them, however, public health nurses could not hold the central place within the health care system that had once, albeit briefly, been theirs. As medical interest shifted away from problems of infection and public interest in the health of the poor declined, the concerns of public health nurses became less and less widely shared.[33]

Thus, turn-of-the-century America witnessed a special moment in the history of public health nursing. Unique social, medical, and economic realities all combined to create a demand for a new kind of worker who could care for the sick poor and working classes in their homes. The trained nurse seemed the perfect solution to a set of complex and interrelated problems. Public health nursing had considerable symbolic and practical appeal and offered nurses an irresistible combination—economic security and professional independence.

Developing under the aegis of a variety of disparate and different private and public agencies, however, public health nursing never generated the kinds of structures that might have enabled public health nurses to establish themselves as a cohesive, recognized, and powerful group within the health care system. Although nurses did help to bring about some changes within the domain of public health, this field's development was determined predominantly by factors beyond the control of organized nursing. Quite logically, therefore, as circumstances began to change the medical care system in the late 1920s, public health nurses found themselves responding to the outcome, rather than shaping what that outcome would be.

Within the fee-for-service hospital-based system of medical care that has become increasingly entrenched since the 1920s, the work of the public health nurse has continued to decline in significance. During the optimistic years before World War I, it would have been difficult to believe that the public health nurse would play such a marginal role. And yet, in retrospect, it is unfortunately clear that the growth and promise of public health nursing at that time was little more than a false dawn.

NOTES

Support from the American Nurses' Foundation Nurses' Educational Funds, Inc. and the Division of Nursing, Department of Health and Human Services, grant #NU-05087 made this research possible. The author wishes to thank the following for their comments on earlier drafts: Maurie Kerrigan, Susan Reverby, Charles Rosenberg, Judy Smith, and Morris Vogel.

1. The quotation by Winslow is from C.-E. A. Winslow, "Public Health Nursing," quoted in Allen Albert, "Nursing as a Social Influence," *American Journal of Nursing* (hereafter cited as *AJN*) 36 (May 1936): 490.

2. Charles Rosenberg, "Social Class and Medical Care in 19th Century America: The Rise and Fall of the Dispensary," *Journal of the History of Medicine* 29 (January 1974): 32–54; George Rosen, "The First Neighborhood Health Center Movement—Its Rise and Fall," *American Journal of Public Health* 61 (August 1971): 1620–35; Morris Vogel, "The Transformation of the American Hospital, 1850–1920," in *Health Care in America: Essays in Social History*, ed. Susan Reverby and David Rosner (Philadelphia: Temple University Press, 1979), pp. 105–16; and David Rosner, "Business at the Bedside: Health Care in Brooklyn, 1890–1915," in *Health Care in America*, pp. 117–31.

3. Rosenberg, "Social Class and Medical Care," and Rosen, "First Neighborhood Health Center Movement." Visiting nurses were not alone in this respect, health centers and dispensaries shared a similar fate.

4. Harriet Fulmer, "History of Visiting Nurse Work in America," *AJN* 2 (March 1902): 411–25.

5. For a discussion of these ideas see ibid.; Mary Beard, "Home Nursing," *Public Health Nurse Quarterly* (hereafter cited as *PHNQ*) 7 (January 1915): 44–57; Annie Brainard, *The Evolution of Public Health Nursing* (Philadelphia: Saunders Co., 1922), p. 211; Visiting Nurse Association of Providence, *Annual Report of 1908* (Providence, 1908), p. 20. The story is quoted from Visiting Nurse Association of Providence, *Annual Report of 1907* (Providence, 1907), p. 29.

6. For an early discussion of the economic importance of these nurses, see Fulmer, "History of Visiting Nurse Work in America," p. 412. For a fuller discussion of the changing economic needs of hospitals, see Vogel, "The Transformation of the American Hospital," pp. 105–16; Rosner, "Business at the Bedside," pp. 117–31; and "The Hospital Deficit," *Trained Nurse and Hospital Review* 32 (February 1904): 115, editorial.

7. Mary Gardner is quoted from Mary Gardner, "Twenty-Five Years Ago," *Public Health Nurse* (hereafter cited as *PHN*) 29 (March 1937): 142. The origins of the Metropolitan Life Insurance Company (MLI) nursing programs are described in Ella Crandall, "Memoranda on Circumstances Leading to the Organization of the National Organization for Public Health Nursing," May 1921, Gardner Papers, folder 45, Schlesinger Library, Radcliffe College, Cambridge, Mass. (hereafter cited as Gardner, "Memoranda"); Metropolitan Life Insurance Company, *The Welfare Work of Metropolitan Life Insurance for Its Industrial Policyholders; Report 1915* (New York: MLI, 1915), p. 3; Lee Frankel, *Visiting Nursing and Life Insurance: A Statistical Summary of Results of Eight Years* (New York: MLI, June 1918), p. 2; *Intelligencer*, MLI 5–6 (September 1911), p. 4; and Ella Crandall, "A New Extension of Visiting Nursing," *AJN* 10 (January 1909): 236–39.

8. Josephine Goldmark, *Nursing and Nursing Education in the United States* (New York: Macmillan, 1923), p. 42; and Yssabella Waters, *Visiting Nursing in the United States* (New York: Charties Publication, 1909), pp. 340–45.

9. Quotations are from Beard, "Home Nursing," pp. 45–47; Brainard, *Evolution*, pp. 323–326; and Mary Gardner, *Public Health Nursing* (New York: Macmillan, 1916), pp. 29–30.

10. The quotation is from Isabel Lowman, "The Need of a Standard for Visiting Nursing," *Visiting Nurse Quarterly* (hereafter cited as *VNQ*) 4 (January 1912): p. 14. For a detailed description of the Metropolitan Life Insurance Co. situation, see Gardner, "Memoranda." The company's service had been organized in 1909 as a strictly graduate nurse program in accordance with the standards for the work stipulated by Wald. Ella Crandall had organized the nursing service for Metropolitan Life Insurance Company before becoming an instructor at Teachers College, Columbia. Eleanor Mumford, "Field Interview with Ella Phillips Crandall," Jan. 19, 1937, Gardner Papers, folder 45, Schlesinger Library, Radcliffe College, Cambridge, Mass. In one of the associations approached by Frankel, the company had

paid for 33,494 visits that year. See Grace Allison, "Shall Attendants Be Trained and Registered?" *AJN* 12 (August 1912), p. 933.

11. Wald, Foley, and Crandall discussed the matter with Frankel, reminding him of the terms and conditions stipulated by Wald when the service was initiated. To these nurses the company's action seemed to indicate a serious tendency toward commercialism. Gardner, "Memoranda." Foley's quotation is from Edna Foley, "Concerning the Employing of Practical Nurses by Visiting Nurse Associations" *AJN* 12 (January 1912): 328, 330.

12. For the Goodrich quotation, see Annie Goodrich, "The Need for Orientation," *AJN* 13 (February 1913): 341.

13. After initiating this program around 1913, the company was able to reduce the number of visits to chronic cases by over twenty thousand each year. *The Welfare Work of Metropolitan Life Insurance Company for Its Industrial Policyholders; Report 1915* (New York: MLI, 1915), p. 3. Isabel Lowman's quotation is from Lowman, "The Need of a Standard," p. 15.

14. Committee members from the American Nurses' Association were Jane Delano, Anna Kerr, and Ella Crandall; from the Superintendents Society they were Edna Foley, Mary Gardner, and Mary Beard. All were public health nurses. See "Report of the Joint Committee Appointed for Consideration of the Standardization of Visiting Nursing," *Proceedings of 18th Annual Convention of the American Society of Superintendents of Training Schools for Nurses* (Springfield, Mass.: Thatcher Art Printery, 1912), pp. 118–24. See also the discussion of establishment of National Organization for Public Health Nursing in M. Louise Fitzpatrick, *The National Organization for Public Health Nursing, 1912–1952: Development of a Practice Field* (New York: National League for Nursing, 1975), pp. 20–36 (hereafter cited as Fitzpatrick, *NOPHN*). Crandall is quoted from Brainard, *Evolution*, p. 334. The discussion leading to this decision is presented in "The 15th National Convention of American Nurses' Association," *VNQ* 4 (July 1912): 43–68.

15. Winslow is quoted from C.-E. A. Winslow, "The Untilled Fields of Public Health," *Science* 51 (January 1920), p. 6. For further discussion of this new role, see C.-E. A. Winslow, "The New Profession of Public Health Nursing and Its Educational Needs," speech, 1917, p. 4, Winslow Collection, folder 119:128, Yale University Library, New Haven, Conn. (hereafter cited as Winslow Collection); and Goldmark, *Nursing*, pp. 7, 128–29. The medical authority is quoted from *Their Health Is Your Health*, fund-raising booklet for Henry Street Nurses' Settlement, 1934.

16. For example, see Visiting Nurse Association of Providence, *Annual Report* (1906–7). These reports support the idea that with specialty work, actual "nursing care" was of course, not possible for the nurse. See Edna Foley, "The Past and Future of the Tuberculosis Nurse," *National Association for Study and Prevention of Tuberculosis*, Proceedings, Seventh Annual Meeting (Chicago, 1911), p. 122; Brainard, *Evolution*, p. 420; and

Mary Beard, "Generalization in Public Health Nursing," *PHNQ* 5 (October 1913): 42–47.

17. See, for example, H. W. Hill, "Is the Visiting Nurse a Public Health Nurse?" *PHN* 11 (July 1919): 486–88, and Bessie Haasis, "Public Health Nursing, An Agent of Americanization," *PHN* 11 (July 1919): 493–96. Davis is quoted from Michael Davis, *Immigrant Health and the Community* (New York: Harper and Brothers, 1921), p. 379.

18. Isabel Stewart, "Readjustment of Our Training School Curriculum to Meet the New Demands of Public Health Nursing," *AJN* 19 (November 1919): 102–9; and Brainard, *Evolution*, p. 317.

19. Crowell is quoted from "The 15th National Convention of the American Nurses' Association," *VNQ* 4 (July 1912): 49. See Fitzpatrick, *NOPHN*, pp. 48–53, 70–72, for a discussion of these activities.

20. This was not an original solution. Emerson's new worker was modeled after the role of the English health visitor. S. O. Baker to Haven Emerson, Dec. 17, 1918, Nutting Papers, "health visitor" folder, Department of Nursing Education Archives, Teachers College, Columbia University, New York (hereafter cited as MAN).

21. See the letters written by nursing leadership in response to Emerson's proposal in "health visitor" folder, MAN collection. The Emerson quotation can be found in Haven Emerson to M. Adelaide Nutting, Aug. 1, 1917, "health visitor" folder, MAN collection. The new role and salary are discussed in M. Adelaide Nutting, Memorandum on Training for Health Visitors, July 13, 1917, "health visitor" folder, MAN collection. To put the smallness of this salary into perspective, it should be noted that in 1909 the Health Department was paying nurses $900–$1200 per year. Waters, *Visiting Nursing*, p. 341.

22. J. A. Duffy, *A History of Public Health in New York City: 1866–1966* (New York: Russell Sage, 1974), p. 276, mentions Emerson's removal from office. For a more detailed discussion of these various plans, see E. V. Brumbaugh, "Public Health Instructor, A New Type of Health Worker," *American Journal of Public Health* (hereafter cited as *AJPH*) 18 (September 1918): 662–64; Agnes Randolph, "The New Law in Virginia," *PHNQ* 10 (July 1918): 295–301; and Portia Kernodle, *The Red Cross Nurse in Action: 1882–1948* (New York: Harper & Brothers, 1949), pp. 166–78.

23. Dr. Robertson presented his plan in John Dill Robertson, "Who Shall Nurse the Sick?" *AJPH* 11 (January 1921): 108–12. The story of the nurse is quoted from Amy Hillard, "A Discussion of the Report of the Rockefeller Committee and Its Effect in Practice Upon the Hospital Nursing Department" in *Transactions of the American Hospital Association, 24th Annual Convention* (Chicago, 1922), p. 182.

24. The nurse from Virginia is quoted from Randolph, "The New Law in Virginia," p. 296. Vincent's views are discussed in a letter from Ella Crandall to C.-E. A. Winslow, Nov. 21, 1918, folder 86:1390, Winslow Collection. See also Fitzpatrick, *NOPHN*, pp. 72–76; and T. E. Christy,

et al., "An Appraisal of *An Abstract for Action*," in Florence Downs and Margaret Newman, *A Source Book of Nursing Research* (Philadelphia: F. A. Davis Co., 1973), p. 230.

25. Randolph, "The New Law in Virginia," p. 297.

26. Fitzpatrick, *NOPHN*, p. 70; and "Code for Aid and Attendant Service Under Public Health Nursing Agencies," *PHNQ* 10 (July 1918): 302; Mary Beard, "The Attendant as an Assistant to Public Health Nurses," *PHN* 11 (March 1919): 181–83; Florence Caldwell, "The Attendant as an Assistant to Public Health Nurses," *PHN* 11 (May 1919): 346; Dorothy Deming, *The Practical Nurse* (New York: Commonwealth Fund, 1947), p. 164; and Blanche Swainhart, "The Supervised Attendant Service," *PHNQ* 10 (April 1918): 183–98.

27. George Vincent to Adelaide Nutting, Dec. 4, 1918, Goldmark folder, MAN collection. For questions of interest to the Foundation, see History 900–02, Source Material Vol. 8, pp. 2089–90, Rockefeller Foundation Archives, North Tarrytown, New York. For correspondence and minutes of the committee see Goldmark folder, MAN collection.

28. Hillard, "A Discussion of the Report of the Rockefeller Committee," p. 182. The committee's recommendations are quoted from Goldmark, *Nursing*, pp. 10–11, 14–15. See also Mary Beard, "Discussion of Goldmark Report," *Proceedings of the 29th Annual Convention of the National League for Nursing Education* (Baltimore: Williams & Wilkins, 1923), p. 184.

29. Winslow reviews the definition of public health nursing in current use in a letter, C.-E. A. Winslow to Mathilda Kuhlman, March 4, 1926, folder 61:711, Winslow Collection. The new NOPHN definition can be found in Fitzpatrick, *NOPHN*, p. 102. The quotation of Winslow is from Winslow, "The New Profession of Public Health Nursing." The most desirable way to organize the work of public health nurses was through a generalized nursing service whereby all nursing care—preventive and curative, public and private—was administered by a single agency with each nurse being responsible for all cases within her district. This organizational solution was supported by the Goldmark Report and the East Harlem Study, but by 1931 only 2 percent of all agencies were under such a combined administration. Goldmark, *Nursing*, pp. 8–10; and East Harlem Nursing and Health Service, *A Comparative Study of Generalized and Specialized Health Services* (New York: East Harlem Nursing and Health Service, 1926). Louise Tattershall, "Census of Public Health Nursing in the United States, 1931," *PHN* 24 (April 1932): 206.

30. For a further discussion of these changes, see Judith Walzer Leavitt and Ronald L. Numbers, "Sickness and Health in America: An Overview," in *Sickness and Health in America*, ed. Judith Leavitt and Ronald Numbers (Madison: University of Wisconsin Press, 1978), pp. 3–10; Gretchen Condran and Rose Cheney, "Mortality Trends in Philadelphia: Age and Cause-Specific Death Rates 1870–1930," paper presented at Annual

Meeting of the Population Association of America, Denver, 1980; Rosen, "The First Neighborhood Health Center Movement," 1620–35; and Vogel, "The Transformation of the American Hospital," pp. 110–14. For a discussion of the growth of the hospital, see "Hospital Service in the United States," *Journal of the American Medical Association* 100 (March 1933): 887.

31.   For data describing the numbers of public health nurses, see Coldmark, *Nursing*, p. 42; Louise Tattershall, "Census of Public Health Nursing in the United States," *PHN* 18 (May 1926): 263; and Louise Tattershall, *Public Health Nursing in the United States: January 15, 1931* (New York: National Organization for Public Health Nursing, 1931). Gardner, *Public Health Nursing*, pp. 154, 430–31. The Boston Association, Instructive District Nursing Association, later Community Health Association, began to have problems raising sufficient funds in the 1920s. By 1923 they were considering limitations on the intake of work and finally their "hard" financial problems forced them to reduce the annual budget by $130,000. See, for example, Minutes of the Board of Managers 1920, Supervisor Meeting Book 1923, Board of Managers 1923, and Board of Managers Minutes for 1924. In 1931, only 36 percent of public health agencies were voluntary; by 1979 they had decreased to 5 percent. See Tattershall, "Census of Public Health Nursing in the United States, 1931," p. 206; and U.S. Department of Health and Human Services, Health Resources Administration, Division of Nursing, 1979 Survey of Community Health Nursing, unpublished data, Washington, D.C. Louise Tattershall, "Hourly Nursing in Public Health Nursing Associations," *PHN* 19 (August 1927): 397–402.

32.   National Organization for Public Health Nursing, *Survey of Public Health Nursing: Administration and Practice* (New York: Commonwealth Fund, 1934), pp. 28–31.

33.   Ibid. By 1931, 63 percent of all agencies and 61 percent of all public health nurses were employed under official auspices. See Tattershall, *Census*, p. 3. This fate was shared with physicians interested in public health. See George Rosen, *Preventive Medicine in the United States, 1900–1975: Trends and Interpretations* (New York: Prodist, 1977), pp. 52–54.

6

The Silent Battle:
Nurse Registration in New York State,
1903–1920

Nancy Tomes

State regulation, as historians and sociologists have long recognized, played a pivotal part in the twentieth-century rise of the professions. The restrictive licensing laws passed in the late 1800s strengthened the professions not simply by granting them legal monopolies over the provision of certain services, but also by extending their powers of self-regulation. The establishment of state licensing boards, whose members were selected from official professional societies and delegated the authority to examine and license practitioners, enabled the most powerful elements within a field to exclude competitors and develop more uniform intellectual and ethical codes. Standardizing and limiting access to professional practice in turn enhanced its social and economic rewards. As Eliot Friedson has argued in his influential study of the medical profession, it has been this autonomy, or privilege of self-regulation and evaluation, that more than any other factor has distinguished the professions from the skilled trades. Somewhat paradoxically, then, increasing state regulation has made a fundamental contribution to the modern-day prestige of the professions.[1]

The importance of state regulation in creating a stronger profession can nowhere be better documented than for the field of medicine. Numerous scholars have examined the period from 1890 to 1920, a period during which the passage of new medical practice acts gave unprecedented power to the "regular" physicians represented by the state medical societies. The societies' control over the state boards of medical examiners, which gained sole authority for licensure during the Progressive era, facilitated changes in medical education long envisioned by reformers as an antidote to the nineteenth-century physician's low status and financial insecurity. By making licensing dependent upon the candidate's educational credentials as well as passage of a qualifying examination, the state boards forced medical schools to adopt higher preliminary education requirements and substantial curriculum changes. State regulation proved especially useful in limiting the growth of competing medical sects, such as osteopathy and chiropractic, since the "regular" physicians on the licensing boards could make it difficult for "irregular" schools to gain state recognition and could devise qualifying exams that sectarian physicians found hard to pass. Aided by the American Medical Association and corporate philanthropies such as the Rockefeller and Carnegie Foundations, the licensing boards worked to reduce the number of medical schools and medical practitioners. The 1910 Flexner Report, which advocated abolishing many medical schools and upgrading the rest, only strengthened a movement already underway at the state level. By the 1910s physicians had successfully used medical licensing laws to advance their social and economic position.[2]

The history of the medical profession obviously supports the contention that restrictive licensing laws have promoted occupational autonomy and prestige. Without denying that this premise has much validity, however, it is essential to examine the development of other skilled fields, to see if state regulation has necessarily had the same effect in every case. Too often sociological concepts of professionalization have been based exclusively upon medicine. Only by comparative study of the professions can the tendency toward oversimplified models of professional development be overcome. To this end the history of nursing, as a predominantly female occupation closely allied to medicine, yet perceived as far less autonomous and prestigious, provides a useful corrective. More specifically, the history of the nurse registration movement allows a closer examination of the prevailing formulations concerning licensure and professional autonomy.[3]

In comparison to the well-documented saga of the medical "move toward monopoly," professional nursing's attempt to achieve a similar revolution in status during the same period has gone virtually unnoticed by general historians. The nurse registration movement, like other facets of nursing's past, has until recently been of interest only to nurses themselves. Historical analysis of registration has gone little beyond the first inspirational accounts written by the movement's leaders. Traditional nursing history has tended to accept the early leadership's protestations of "disinterested benevolence" in championing registration, without acknowledging the ways in which protective legislation favored the leaders' own self-interests. By relying on favorable accounts of the measure, nurse historians have minimized opposition to registration and perpetuated the assumption that the reform achieved all that its advocates claimed for it. More particularly, the emphasis on the initial passage of the state laws, without any consideration of their varying provisions or subsequent administration, has obscured the real impact of the registration movement. To date, nursing history has only reinforced the notion that the mere acquisition of licensing laws in and of itself is sufficient to establish a profession's credibility. But as the example of nurse registration so well demonstrates, this assumption proves to be far from true.[4]

In reassessing the significance of the registration movement, we would do well to recall a comment made by Lavinia Dock, one of nursing's first (and best) historians: "Restrictive legislation . . . is not to be gained once and forever. . . . It does not mean just one effort but continuous efforts for the rest of time," she wrote in 1900. Heeding Dock's insight, this study will examine the administration of New York State's first nurse registration bill. From reports published by the state's nurse examiners, and accounts (both favorable and unfavorable) in contemporary professional journals, this paper will assess registration's impact on New York's nursing schools and nurses. What such a case-study approach loses in generality will be more than compensated for by the complex understanding of professional politics that it provides. In particular, by comparing the outcome of the New York nurses' legislative efforts with the medical reform occurring in the same time period, we can gain new insight into the ways gender and institutional relationships affected professionalization.[5]

The nurses' registration movement grew out of a sense of professional crisis very similar to that felt by late nineteenth-century medical men. Although a comparatively young vocation, first introduced in the United States during the 1870s, trained nursing grew so rapidly that by 1900, problems of "overproduction" and lack of standardization had already begun to vex its professional leaders. The increasing complexity of medical technology and the simultaneous proliferation of hospitals stimulated the expansion of the training-school system as a cheap but efficient means to meet the labor demands of the new scientific medicine. At the same time the growing appreciation of medical care among the rising middle class increased the need for private duty nurses. In addition to hospital schools, many commercial and correspondence schools of nursing sprang up to fulfill this demand. Needless to say, the preparation offered by the various institutions differed widely in length and scope, from the three-year hospital school programs to the short-term correspondence courses. By the turn of the century the term "trained nurse" had come to cover a wide variety of practitioners, from the elite alumnae of the Johns Hopkins Training School to the numerous graduates of the Chautauqua Correspondence School of Nursing. To further confuse the public, the ranks of "untrained" or "natural" nurses, particularly midwives, continued to grow along with the massive waves of immigration. The 1900 census listed a mere 12,000 "graduate" or "trained" nurses to 109,000 "untrained" nurses and midwives.[6]

The hospital-based nursing elite, women like Isabel Hampton and Adelaide Nutting of the Johns Hopkins School of Nursing, viewed with concern both the lack of uniformity among trained nurses and the multiplicity of their untrained competitors. By the early 1900s these nursing leaders had become convinced that state regulation represented the one best means to impose order on a chaotic, overcrowded field. A law requiring nurses to be registered by the state would give nursing leaders a centralized source of power with which to regulate the whole profession. Nurse boards of examiners, exactly like those established by the medical societies, could be used to enforce standards that would distinguish the "real" trained nurse from her unqualified competitors. Thus between 1900 and 1920 acquisition of licensing laws dominated the profession's political agenda; by 1923 state nurses' societies, formed expressly to win registration laws, had secured some type of regulation in all forty-eight states.[7]

New York State's legislative effort played a key role in the national registration movement for several reasons. In the early twentieth century New York was the undisputed nursing capital of the United States, with more nurses and training schools than any other state. Not only their numbers but also their level of organization gave New York nurses a national leadership role. The New York State Nurses Association (NYSNA), founded in 1901, was the first state society formed in the country. While not the first passed, the registration bill the NYSNA secured was certainly the most restrictive of the early state laws, and therefore closest to the professional leaders' concept of the "ideal" legislation. The national prominence of several nurses involved in administering New York's law, including Sophia Palmer, the influential editor of the *American Journal of Nursing*, and Annie Goodrich, a prominent young training school superintendent, focused further attention on New York developments. Thus the regulatory efforts of the New York Board of Nurse Examiners received close national scrutiny. As Charlotte Aikens, a critic of the registration movement, remarked in the *Trained Nurse and Hospital Review* in 1909, New York had become the "central source of registration wisdom" and nurses in other states measured their gains against the Empire State's achievements.[8]

The "power" of the New York bill, as its admirers frequently pointed out, stemmed from its administration by the Board of Regents, a government agency created in 1784 to supervise higher education in the state. From the 1870s on, the Regents had gradually acquired responsibility for the regulation of various professional groups, including physicians, dentists, veterinarians, and accountants. The authority to certify both the individual practitioner *and* the educational institution had made the board a powerful agent for professional regulation. The Regents did not confine themselves solely to licensing professionals, but also had to approve the schools where the aspiring candidates received their training. The Education Department's *Annual Report* for 1904 stated that the Regents aimed at nothing less than "to bring to a uniformly high standard the various institutions of the state, to protect the public from illegal and inexperienced practitioners, and incidentally to raise the standard in other states." In medicine's case, for example, the Regents' assumption in 1890 of all licensing authority had facilitated the reform of the state's medical schools and helped to stem the growth of sectarian medicine. By 1900 the Regents' advocacy of professional regulation through educational reform had placed New York's Board of Medical Examiners at the forefront of the national reform movement.[9]

In drafting their bill, the NYSNA relied heavily upon the experience and advice of the medical men allied with the Regents Office. The 1903 nurses' legislation merely copied the administrative structure already used by the board to regulate the medical profession. The law authorized the Regents to select a Nurse Board of Examiners from a list submitted by the NYSNA. These examiners had the power (subject to the Regents' approval, of course) to determine (1) the level of preliminary education required of students entering the training school; (2) the minimum requirements for a nursing education; (3) the scope and evaluation of the qualifying examination; and (4) the process of registering nurses. Furthermore, the bill specified that even to sit for the examination, a candidate had to be a graduate of at least a two-year program offered at a school registered by the Regents "as maintaining . . . proper standards." Together the nurse examiners and the Regents were to decide exactly what constituted these "proper standards."[10]

The nurses' registration bill differed from the legislation regulating medicine in only one crucial respect: compliance remained a voluntary rather than a mandatory requirement. A nurse had to meet the Regents' standards in order to use the title "Registered Nurse," but need not be registered in order to practice nursing. In other words the 1903 law prohibited no one from nursing for hire, whatever his or her qualifications; it guaranteed only that those practitioners identifying themselves as "R.N.s" had met the state's standards. In New York the same limitation applied to the title "certified public accountant," but not to the terms "physician," "dentist," or "veterinarian." Because the latter fields were governed by a mandatory law, no practitioner could claim to practice medicine, dentistry, or veterinarian medicine unless licensed by the Regents. While the NYSNA certainly wanted nursing to be protected by the same legal restriction, it recognized that nurses did not have the political power in 1903 to achieve a mandatory law, and settled for as restrictive a voluntary statute as could be obtained.[11]

Despite its limited scope, the NYSNA's 1903 bill met with considerable opposition because it made registration contingent upon certain educational requirements. Sizable factions among both nursing and medical practitioners believed that registration should be made a simple matter of signing up at the Regents' Office, not a test of an individual's educational achievement or an institution's academic program. The NYSNA, the opposition argued, did not represent the field as a whole, and would invariably set licensing standards that discriminated against the vast majority of nurses. In addition the medical proprietors of small private hospital schools protested that they would be the victims of unfair regulation. Registration's critics concluded that the "reforms" enacted by the NYSNA and the Regents would in effect be "special-interest" legislation, favorable only to "higher education enthusiasts" and hospital nurses.[12]

The registration bill passed in spite of these objections primarily because the Regents, the state medical establishment, and several large New York City hospitals backed the more restrictive model of legislation. The Regents argued that the trained nurse should be accorded the same protective regulation extended to other professionals; to question that position implicitly challenged the basic premise of the Regents' authority. The state medical society, having fought its own legislative battles over the right to exclusive representation of the medical profession, proved sympathetic to the NYSNA's political aspirations. Within the medical profession as a whole, progressive physicians, especially the "hospital men," approved registration as a method of securing a more "reliable assistant and invaluable associate." The prospect of driving the small private or "special" hospitals out of business by the "rigid exclusion" of their training schools from state recognition had additional appeal. The lay managers and superintendents of the influential New York City hospitals supported registration for much the same reasons doctors backed the reform. Both these factions saw that the regulation of nursing could further scientific medicine and hospital efficiency, the two central goals of Progressive-era medicine. Thus "liberal-minded" elements within New York's educational, medical, and hospital establishments endorsed the 1903 bill because it furthered their interests, along with those of the NYSNA.[13]

In many respects the administration of the new registration act over the next decade fulfilled its opponents' worst fears, as well as outstripped some of its supporters' expectations. The Nurse Board of Examiners appointed in 1903, the Inspector of Training Schools hired in 1906, and the Nurse Advisory Council, a policy-setting group set up in 1907, formed a powerful lobby for educational reform. The nurses who served in these positions during the early years of registration believed wholeheartedly in "the upbuilding of the schools . . . through the state," as Annie Goodrich expressed it. Sophia Palmer, the first president of the Board of Examiners, frequently stated that the Regents had given nurses the power to set their "lines," or standards; slowly over the years those lines would be "drawn in" to pull the "lower-grade" schools up to an acceptable level. Due to registration "we are going to get from year to year a little better education, a little broader education, and a little more thorough education for the nurses throughout New York State," concluded Palmer.[14]

The nurses' ambitions did not stop with their own state. The Regents' authority to register out-of-state schools gave the New York legislation a "reflex influence" much prized by its admirers. Since so many trained nurses came to the state to practice, nursing leaders realized that the "power" of this one registration act could be used to standardize and upgrade nursing schools throughout the country. The New York law inspired ambitious plans for affiliation, reciprocity, even a national board of examiners. Thus when the first New York State Board of Nurse Examiners gathered in 1904 to set the initial Regents' rules for nursing schools, its members self-consciously aimed at a "universal standard" that would assist all high-minded educational reformers in their "one silent battle" to improve the profession. Following the lead of the medical reformers, the nursing elite planned to make state-mandated educational reform the cornerstone of their program for professional uplift.[15]

The Nurse Board of Examiners' first guidelines, which went into effect between 1904 and 1906, were indeed comprehensive. The Regents' rules stipulated first that no hospital with less than twenty-five beds could have an approved training school. A minimum of two, preferably three, years of instruction had to be provided; in addition probationers were to receive at least two weeks, preferably one to six months, of preliminary instruction before beginning ward work. Hospitals having a three-year program could use their senior pupils for private duty work for no more than three months. Finally, every school's curriculum had to provide "practical" (i.e., ward) and "theoretical" (i.e., classroom) work in five basic nursing areas: medical, surgical, obstetrical, children's, and dietetics. In addition some theoretical training had to be given in the care of contagious diseases.[16]

Despite Sophia Palmer's assertion that the state's hospital schools would not be "unjustly demoralized" by these "very simple" requirements, the majority of institutions could not initially meet the Regents' standards. The examiners had set the requisites well below those of the leading training schools such as Presbyterian and St. Luke's in New York City. But as the nurses well knew, practices in the vast majority of schools bore little resemblance to the standards in the leading city hospitals. Only nineteen of New York State's ninety-eight incorporated schools found that they could meet the Regents' rules without making changes in their operation. Among the rest, the registration act almost immediately began to produce "a sort of stir," as Palmer noted happily.[17]

The major impact of the examiners' initial standards centered on the basic curriculum requirements. Although 60 percent of the schools operating in 1904 already had a three-year course, only a third could provide the "rounded" training demanded by the Regents. Most so-called "general" hospitals in the state had no maternity or pediatric wards, for example. Registration set off a scramble to add special wards or form affiliations with the small maternity and children's hospitals. By 1907 almost 50 percent of the training schools had formed affiliations in order to meet the state requirements.[18]

Probably the most dramatic realignment brought about by the first Regents' guidelines could be seen in the training schools run by the state's mental hospitals. In order to make their graduates eligible for registration, the Lunacy Commission had to bargain long and hard with the Nurse Board of Examiners. The examiners considered the curriculum and supervision of these schools so inferior that they at first resisted yielding "in any point" to accommodate them. But after several years of intense negotiation with the Lunacy Commission, the examiners approved compromises on the standards required of the state hospitals that allowed their training schools to be approved and to send graduates to the exam. In exchange each accredited state school had to hire a nurse trained in a general hospital to serve as superintendent of nursing, a post hitherto nonexistent in the asylum's administrative structure, and had to form affiliations to provide pediatric and maternity experience in the third year. In a very tentative way, the examiners began to force some convergence between the nursing schools run by two very different types of hospitals. Even this limited movement toward standardization cost a high price, for in later years the Lunacy Commission would prove to be a powerful opponent of the Nurse Examiners.[19]

The dislocations caused by the 1904/1906 regulations did not immediately concern the Nurse Examiners, however. Instead they hailed the "stirrings" produced by the guidelines as a sign of success, and tried to prolong their unsettling effect. Between 1906 and 1911, the Regents Office nurses continually expanded and refined their supervisory powers. To see how closely institutions conformed to the statutory requirements, the inspector of training schools began to demand written reports from the superintendents and paid periodic visits to each school, to observe "actual conditions" and suggest "adjustment of details" to make the training "conform more nearly to regulations," as Anna Alline, the first inspector, wrote. The information collected by the inspector in turn enabled the examiners and the Advisory Council to generate new policies. In response to the superintendents' repeated requests for curriculum suggestions, for example, the examiners published a "Course of Study and Syllabus" in 1906, which outlined the topics a student would have to master in order to pass the qualifying exam. Discovering that almost a third of the state's nursing schools had no assistant superintendent to supervise the ward and classroom work called for by the suggested curriculum, the examiners lobbied for more assistants; by 1911 the percentage of schools without such an officer had dropped to 9 percent. In like fashion, the Regents Office nurses linked every reform they advocated with successful completion of the registration exam; in their propaganda shorter work hours, better living conditions, more hired lecturers, in fact all desirable changes, were presented as means to this ultimate goal.[20]

Unfortunately for their purposes the examiners' ambitions often overreached their regulatory authority. By law they had no power to implement reforms beyond the minimum specified in the official regulations, namely, those covering the number of beds, requisite topics, length of program, and preliminary educational requirements. So while the Regents' rules stated what topics had to be taught, they did not stipulate the manner or length of each subject's presentation. While correcting this deficiency, the examiners' syllabus remained only a recommended, not a required, outline. As a result, Annie Goodrich, upon assuming the inspector's post in 1911, found tremendous variation in the approved schools' curricula. The amount of work devoted to dietetics, for example, ranged from two to sixty-four lectures a year. Overall very few programs met all the criteria set forth in the examiners' syllabus. Grading the registered schools against her ideal, Goodrich gave only two institutions an excellent rating, and twenty an "above average" mark. The vast majority, eighty-two schools, met only the minimum requirements; ten institutions did not even achieve that minimum. Clearly the examiners' ability to implement any standards beyond the baseline set by law was very circumscribed.[21]

Still, by 1911 the nursing elite had established a not inconsiderable base of administrative power in the Regents' office. The Nurse Examiners had enforced a set of minimum standards and developed a regular supervisory routine. While institutions might evade specific reforms endorsed by the Regents Office nurses, they could not escape the nurses' observation and intrusion. The inspector of training schools had to make her visits, the reports to the Regents had to be filed, and the directives from Albany had to be read. Welcome or not, the examiners and their associates had become a persistent presence in the state's training schools.

Moreover the examiners were in an excellent position slowly to expand their presence. Whatever difficulties they had encountered in urging voluntary reform, the nursing leadership had discovered two potent means to advance their cause. First, their control over the contents of the registration exam ensured that any school wanting its graduates to make a good showing had to pay some heed to the examiners' curriculum suggestions. In practical terms a school that slighted dietetics or chemistry too thoroughly ran the risk of seeing its candidates fail those sections of the test. Second, the examiners had built a close working relationship with the Regents and the first assistant commissioner of education, Augustus Downing, who had immediate authority over the nursing office. On a day-to-day basis the nurses serving in Albany had a far better opportunity to influence policy formation than their isolated, far-removed constituents. Thus the examiners and their allies could continually lobby to see particular reforms turned into state-mandated requirements. While slow in effect their persistent politicking would gradually see the educational standards raised—so the nurses believed.

Until 1911 the examiners managed to implement their goals without provoking the formation of a more powerful lobby to oppose them. During the early years of registration, the nurses confined themselves to changes that discomfited only those hospital schools deviating widely from the standards prevailing in the large urban institutions. The "regular" training schools, as Palmer once referred to the high-quality programs, could meet the Regents' rules with little difficulty. By continually pegging state standards below those schools' practice, the examiners could force standardization at a relatively safe pace. As a 1904 editorial in the *American Journal of Nursing* envisioned, "the higher grade schools will go on broadening and developing, and the lower grade schools, with a uniform, minimum standard, made compulsory, will gradually be brought up to the standards of the advanced schools." The small, "irregular" schools might complain, but their protests carried less political weight than the tacit endorsement of the state's leading hospitals, physicians, and educators.[22]

But this strategy worked only so long as the examiners failed to enforce the one Regents' ruling that the "higher-grade" schools did not wish to obey, the preliminary education requirement. The Regents had ruled that as of 1906 all entering students had to have at least one year of high school or its equivalent. At first the examiners had allowed the training schools either to ignore the requirement or to define its equivalent very loosely. But after the appointment in 1910 of a new inspector of training schools, an ambitious young woman named Annie Goodrich, the standards were strictly enforced. In her new position of authority, Goodrich was determined to see that no student entered nursing school without first meeting the preliminary education requirement.[23]

Goodrich's emphasis on this particular issue stemmed in part from an ambition she shared with many nursing leaders, the desire to attract a "better grade" of women into the field. Demanding a higher level of education seemed one effective way of limiting the number of working- and lower-middle-class applicants, for, in the early twentieth century, high school was still a luxury many young women could not afford. In a more immediate sense, a high preliminary education requirement symbolized professional parity to the nursing leadership. As of 1910 nursing had the lowest entrance standards of all New York State's professional groups. Medical schools, for example, already required four years of high school before matriculation. Thus at two levels the campaign to enforce the one-year-in-high-school ruling came to represent the leadership's efforts to make nursing a more elite, prestigious profession. Since the registration act itself, Goodrich announced in her 1913 annual report, the Regents had taken no more "definitive" step toward placing the training schools "on a sound professional basis" than enforcement of the preliminary education requirement.[24]

Unfortunately some of the 1903 bill's original supporters did not share Annie Goodrich's high opinion of the preliminary education requirement. In January 1912 representatives of New York City's Hospital Conference, an organization of physicians and hospital men devoted to "promoting economy and efficiency in hospital management," met to protest the Regents' action. A petition circulated by the group characterized the one-year-in-high-school ruling as an "impracticable" demand, which would work a "hardship" on the "properly equipped and ethically administered" training schools by limiting their supply of students. The Regents, concluded the petition, had to allow the hospitals a "freer hand" in selecting probationers. In so many words, then, the hospital men made clear their determination that the nursing leadership's hankering for "better-quality" women would not circumvent the hospital's best interests. Support for this position, as manifested by the petition's signatories, came from all the city's major institutions, including Presbyterian, St. Luke's, Postgraduate, New York, and Mount Sinai hospitals.[25]

Stung by this seeming betrayal of their interests by the very "regular" institutions they relied upon most, the Regents Office nurses launched their own vigorous campaign to defend the preliminary education requirement. In her 1913 report Goodrich reprinted the reply to the Hospital Conference petition written by the League of Nursing Education for New York City, a group of reform-minded training-school superintendents. "No school . . . can be considered as ethically conducted which would break down standards which are not excessive, for the purpose of securing a sufficient number of probationers to maintain an unpaid nursing service," the superintendents charged. Hospital men had to be taught that the training school existed primarily as an educational institution, not as a source of cheap labor, they concluded.[26]

In the end the nursing leaders' Albany connections carried the day, for their appeals to educational standards found a receptive audience in the Education Department. Despite the considerable political pressure generated by the hospital lobby, the Regents stood firm behind the examiners' decision. To the educators, the nurses' assessment of the issues at stake in the preliminary requirement controversy seemed the more persuasive. Augustus Downing wrote in 1911 that his experience had convinced him the "commercialization" of nursing schools posed the "greatest obstacle to the effective administration" of the registration law. "The hospital thinks first of its own financial interest and after that of the training of the efficient nurse," he claimed, in language revealingly similar to that employed by Goodrich and her supporters. Demand for student labor could not lead to the lowering of the preliminary education requirement, Downing felt, for "education is a prerequisite to intelligent and efficient nursing.[27]

Thus, with the Regents' support, the examiners won the 1912–13 skirmish over the premilinary education requirement. But the controversy sparked by that issue signaled the beginning of a much broader, more prolonged conflict over the examiners' role in nursing affairs. Between 1913 and 1920 opposition to their policies crystallized around the NYSNA's efforts to convert registration from a voluntary to a mandatory law. The legislative debate over this amendment served to focus the growing resistance to the examiners' administration of the 1903 law. The state's nursing leadership soon found itself confronting a well-organized alliance of critics whose influence even the Regents could not ignore.[28]

Both the NYSNA's efforts to strengthen the registration law's administration and their opponents' attempts to weaken it grew out of the fact that many unregistered graduate nurses were practicing in New York State. As of 1910 registered nurses represented at most 60 percent of the state's graduate nurses. This low figure reflected several developments. In the first place a sizable number of schools had simply decided not to register with the Regents rather than make the changes needed for accreditation. Of the ninety-eight schools listed in the U.S. Bureau of Education's 1904 report, twenty-two, or almost one-third of the total, had not been registered by 1909. Recalcitrant institutions tended to be associated with small, upstate hospitals or staffed by Lutheran or Roman Catholic nursing orders. By 1920 eight of the twenty-two had gone on to gain state approval. Still, a significant minority, roughly 15 percent of the incorporated schools, continued to graduate nurses ineligible to take the registration exam.[29]

More importantly, many nurses actually *eligible* to take the test simply did not bother. In 1911 Annie Goodrich reported that of sixty-nine registered New York schools (60 percent of the state total) who reported the data, twenty-one sent almost the whole graduating class, and thirty-one sent almost half. This showing Goodrich characterized as "the most encouraging" to date. We can only suppose that the schools failing to report these statistics had no better representation at the exam. Not until 1914 did the figures for candidates taking the exam begin to approach the number of diplomas granted by New York State schools; even this convergence was somewhat illusory, for the total number of candidates sitting for the exam included many out-of-state graduates. By whatever measure used, it seems evident that many training schools registered with the Regents did not send their graduates to the exam.[30]

The low turnout for the registration exam suggests that many graduate nurses could find work without possessing the R.N. title. While most forms of institutional nursing, including military, public health, and school service, required registration, the majority of trained nurses did not enter those fields but, rather, went into private duty. Supporters and critics of registration both agreed that the R.N. designation conferred little benefit on the private duty nurse. Neither the average doctor referring jobs to a nurse nor the families interested in hiring her to care for a relative paid much attention to titles; a woman's personal references and training-school affiliation carried much more weight, especially in small towns and rural areas. As a private duty nurse pointed out in a letter to Charlotte Aikens in 1909, "good nurses . . . can get plenty of work without the R.N."[31]

The large percentage of unregistered graduate nurses also reflected the restrictive aim of the original legislation. Neither the NYSNA nor the Nurse Examiners had wanted to make registration easy. On the contrary they had administered the 1903 bill's waiver provisions—which allowed certain categories of nurses already in practice to register without taking the exam—as rigorously as possible. No matter when graduate nurses had taken their training, for example, they could not register under the waiver until their training school met the Regents' requirements then in effect. According to one observer this ruling alone resulted in "arraying hundreds of nurses against the whole movement." Experienced graduates whose schools failed to qualify preferred not to register rather than take the exam on the same footing as the brand-new candidates. The waiver for nurses who lacked any formal education at all, but had extensive "practical experience," proceeded with similar difficulties. The Nurse Examiners insisted on receiving a personal reference from an individual they knew before certifying any such candidate as a "proper person" to be an R.N. Sophia Palmer stated in 1904, "If they are kept waiting ten years they will have to wait, and that is the only way our law is ever going to amount to anything." Finally, the examiners did not prepare an easy qualifying exam. A good many graduates, about 12 percent yearly, simply failed the test. Certain registered schools, the state mental hospitals among them, had such poor records of performance that their students did not even attempt the exam.[32]

Although in many ways a problem of the leadership's own making, the large number of unregistered nurses working in their state greatly concerned the NYSNA and the Regents Office nurses. As the leadership viewed the problem it reflected the limited scope of the original legislation. The 1903 bill had allowed the examiners to register only those trained nurses they felt worthy of the title and to force a minimal upgrading of the registered schools. But because compliance remained voluntary, the law's benefits had not been extended far enough. As long as nursing schools might remain unaccredited and their graduates find work, or as long as eligible nurses could choose to forgo or fail the exam and also find work, so long would registration be limited in its achievements. Given the law's latitude, the "regular" schools would naturally try to flout the Regents' rules they disliked, such as the preliminary education requirements; why obey the examiners when the schools and nurses who ignored them flourished? If "educational standards" were ever to triumph over "hospital economics," the nursing elite reasoned, these loopholes had to be closed. From this line of analysis arose the nurses' determination to pass the NYSNA's amendment, which would restrict the practice of nursing to the R.N. alone. Only by depriving their competitors of the title "nurse" could the truly professional practitioners thrive, so they reasoned.[33]

Opponents of the nursing leaders placed quite a different construction on the same set of circumstances. As the critics viewed it, the large number of unregistered nurses proved that the original bill had been too stringent, not too lenient. If registration's benefits had been made as obvious as the state society alleged, why had so many able women eschewed it? Because, the critics answered, the wrong nurses, the "educational fanatics" bent on their own professional aggrandizement, had administered the act. The examiners and their allies had misused the state's authority to advance their own selfish ends, not the interests of the average nurse or her employer. The Regents had failed to check the nurses' selfish tendencies, due to their own blind commitment to educational reform. One physician wrote that the Regents might be authorities in their own spheres, but they knew nothing about hospitals; "their efforts to apply academic rules to hospital schools have not been and never will be a success," he concluded. As the result, well-intentioned nurses and schools had been saddled with "extreme, impossible" laws.[34]

To extend the nurses' power under the existing terms would be disastrous, opponents of the Regents' policies argued. The Hospital Conference warned hospital superintendents across the state that if the NYSNA's amendment passed, "your training school will be practically governed by this Association." To make registration more than "the little pet scheme" of educators, doctors and hospital men had to have more control over its administration. The Hospital Conference joined the Lunacy Commission, along with the original opponents of registration (the commercial school proprietors and the nurses hostile to the state society) to push alternate legislation. These critics of the NYSNA's amendment agreed unanimously that the all-nurse board of examiners had to be replaced by a "mixed" board of nurses, doctors, and hospital men.[35]

From 1913 on the NYSNA and the Regents-based nurses found themselves fighting not only to extend the scope of registration but also to preserve the administrative power they had so laboriously built up under the original act. In order to achieve mandatory registration over very strong opposition *and* save the all-nurse Board of Examiners, the NYSNA had to make compromise after compromise. First, after two unsuccessful attempts to pass their amendment in 1913 and 1914, the NYSNA allowed the Education Department to take over the bill's sponsorship and tone down its demands. First, the new sponsors changed the act to protect only the terms "trained, graduate, certified or registered" nurse, rather than "nurse," as the NYSNA had first proposed. The bill thus altered again failed to pass the legislature in 1915. In subsequent sessions, more concessions had to be added to win the bill's passage: the reduction of the nurse advisory council from an all-nurse board to one composed of three nurses, three doctors, and three representatives from the incorporated hospitals; provision for the licensing of trained attendants; a generous waiver allowing experienced nurses to register without taking an examination; and a prohibition on any increase in the preliminary education requirement beyond one year of high school until 1930. With all these alterations the mandatory nurse registration bill finally passed the New York State legislature in 1920.[36]

In many respects the 1920 registration bill represented a loss of power for New York State's nursing elite. To gain a mandatory registration law, the NYSNA had to see curtailed much of the autonomy that the early nurse administrators had enjoyed. The new law still retained registration's original "power," that is, the Regents' authority to legislate "proper standards," and preserved the all-nurse Board of Examiners. But in exchange, the nurses had to give up dominance on the policy-making council, to recognize a whole new category of competitors, the trained attendants, and to forgo using what they perceived as the single most effective measure to upgrade nursing's status, the preliminary education requirement. This last compromise was particularly bitter, since the Regents had already agreed as of 1924 to raise the entrance requirement to four years of high school. Taken as a whole these concessions constituted a severe setback to the leadership's effort to limit access to the field and upgrade its prestige. In essence the bill represented one step forward, two steps backward.[37]

The administrative history of New York State's first nurse-practice act suggests that the professional autonomy promised by the 1903 registration act was in fact illusory. The original law passed primarily because it served the purposes of reform factions within medicine and hospital administration. These interest groups saw in registration a means to use nursing as a "hospital yardstick," to borrow historian Susan Reverby's term, on a statewide scale. In other words, by allowing nurses to standardize nursing education, medical reformers could better rationalize and systematize the hospital. Small, unscientific, inefficient institutions would be deprived of their labor force and thereby forced to close or upgrade their standards. So long as registration furthered these goals it retained the support of "liberal-minded" hospital and medical men. For almost the first decade of the act's administration, the nursing elite did indeed promote standardization, as their patrons had hoped. But the nurses' goals in using the law inevitably diverged from the aims of their allies. The leadership's bid for professional parity, particularly the right to limit access to the field, came into conflict with the hospital's need for an abundant labor supply. Once the nurses' interpretation of the law seemed to further their interests at the hospital's expense, the examiners found themselves beset by powerful opponents.[38]

Perhaps if the hospital representatives and the Lunacy Commission had realized in 1903 the "power" even a voluntary law might have, they would have joined the nurses and commercial schools who opposed the original act. As it happened the nursing elite had to demonstrate the power of state regulation before these groups realized its inherent dangers. But rather than dismantle the regulatory machinery already established, the hospital groups simply acquired more efficient means to use the law for their own ends. With permanent representatives on the Advisory Council, medical and hospital concerns in nursing affairs might be more easily advanced. Thus New York State's second nurse-practice act institutionalized a set of conflicting interests that had become well developed over the previous two decades.

In comparison to their medical contemporaries, the nurses' use of the state's licensing power to regulate their field produced far less satisfactory results, at least from the leadership's point of view. During these same decades, nurses had observed the state board of medical examiners and the state medical society engineer a reform of medical education that had restricted access to medical practice and enhanced its prestige.

The physicians too had met opposition, particularly from proprietary medical schools and sectarian doctors, who used arguments similar to those employed against the NYSNA: that the medical society did not represent the majority of physicians; that high educational standards did not necessarily make better doctors; that the Medical Examiners' policies aided only their own selfish interests. Yet in spite of strong resistance the medical leaders had been able to carry through their plan for regulatory reform with considerable success. In light of this example New York's nursing leadership had tried to borrow the "medical model" of professional regulation through educational reform. That their attempts to imitate the medical "move toward monopoly" had far more mixed results must be attributed both to their gender and to their position within the institutional structure of medicine.[39]

Certainly the sex of the occupational groups involved played a central role in determining the outcome of the regulatory process. While autonomy might seem an appropriate goal for a male-dominated profession such as medicine, the "nurses must have entire control" principle, as Charlotte Aikens once termed it, struck many as an unworthy feminine aspiration. Trained nursing had long been justified as an occupation suited for women because of their supposedly inherent traits of self-sacrifice, nurturance, and submissiveness. When professional women acted contrary to the restrictive gender-role prescriptions of their time, they invariably met with more resistance than did men acting in a similar fashion. Parallel to, and reinforcing the gender dimension of the controversy ran the argument over the nurse's place within the institutional hierarchy of medicine. Registration's critics viewed the nurse not as an independent worker, but as the doctor's assistant and the hospital's worker. It seemed only fitting that nurses, as the handmaidens of scientific medicine and hospital efficiency, should set their professional standards subject to the approval of doctors and hospital representatives. The issue of gender became subsumed within a narrower justification for the nurses' subordinate position in the medical hierarchy.[40]

Thus in the early twentieth century medical and hospital interests united to restrain and direct the nurse registration movement for their own ends. While never passive victims of this usurpation, the nursing elite found their power to carry out their own professional agenda severely limited by the interference of other parties. As a result state regulation became not a process whereby one profession governed itself but, rather, a struggle involving three interest groups—four, if the Regents are included—attempting to resolve their conflicting concerns in nursing's affairs. Of course no occupation has ever developed in complete isola-

tion; complex forces have always shaped the process of professionalization, no matter how strong the occupational group involved. Nevertheless some professions have been far more successful than others in
achieving their original aims. The study of licensing laws helps to clarify
the factors that produce this differential level of autonomy. In particular
the history of the registration movement suggests—as might be expected—that the gender of the group involved, and its relationship to
other professions in the field, strongly influence the process of profession-
building.

The status of nursing as a so-called semi-profession, limited in autonomy and prestige, has all too frequently been portrayed as the product
of vague discrimination and impersonal institutional forces. The history
of New York State's registration law reminds us that the restraints
placed upon nurses' autonomy were neither accidental nor unknowing.
As Sophia Palmer once described it, nursing's development reflected a
"silent battle" among several groups involved in its affairs. The same
interests have continued to war with one another up to the time of this
writing. The passage in the New York legislature of the controversial
Laverne-Pisani bill in 1972, which for the first time defined nursing as
distinct from medical practice, represents only the latest, but hardly the
last, episode in an ongoing conflict. So long as nurses, physicians, and
hospitals continue to share the same sphere of professional interests, the
silent battle will not end.[41]

NOTES

My thanks to Ellen Lagemann, Susan Reverby, and Charles Rosenberg for their
editorial comments on this paper.

1.   Older sociological studies of the professions invariably mention the
significance of occupational licensure, although they do not examine the
point in detail. See, for example, A. M. Carr-Saunders, *The Professions:
Their Organization and Place in Society* (Oxford: Clarendon Press, 1933),
esp. pp. 21–26; Ernest Greenwood, "Attributes of a Profession," *Social Work*
2 (July 1957): 48–49; Lee Taylor, *Occupational Sociology* (New York:
Oxford University Press, 1968), esp. pp. 328–29. Newer works, especially
those written from a Marxist perspective, tend to give licensing laws more
emphasis. See, for example, Magali Sarfatti Larson, *The Rise of Professionalism: A Sociological Analysis* (Berkeley: University of California Press,
1977), esp. pp. 14–15.

There is a growing body of specialized literature on contemporary problems concerning state regulation of the professions. See, for example, the re-

cent collection edited by Roger Blair and Stephen Rubin, *Regulating the Professions: A Public Policy Symposium* (Lexington, Mass.: Lexington Books/ D. C. Heath and Co., 1980); the review essay by Marie Haug, "The Sociological Approach to Self-Regulation," pp. 61–80, is especially useful. Little of this new literature has an explicitly historical focus. For the historian's purposes, Lawrence Friedman, "Freedom of Contract and Occupational Licensing, 1890–1910," *California Law Review* 53 (March–May 1965): 487–534, remains the best piece available. J. A. C. Grant, "The Gild Returns to America," *Journal of Politics* 4 (August 1942): 303–36, and 4 (November 1942): 458–77, is a much less systematic, but still interesting review of the same problem.

2. For accounts of the Progressive-era reorganization of medicine, see E. Richard Brown, *Rockefeller Medicine Men* (Berkeley: University of California Press, 1979); James G. Burrow, *Organized Medicine in the Progressive Era* (Baltimore: Johns Hopkins University Press, 1977); William Rothstein, *American Physicians in the Nineteenth Century* (Baltimore: Johns Hopkins University Press, 1972), Richard Shryock, *Medical Licensing in America, 1650–1965* (Baltimore: Johns Hopkins University Press, 1967); Rosemary Stevens, *Medicine and the Public Interest* (New Haven: Yale University Press, 1971); Gerald Markowitz and David Rosner, "Doctors in Crisis," in *Health Care in America: Essays in Social History*, ed. Susan Reverby and David Rosner (Philadelphia: Temple University Press, 1979), pp. 185–205; Robert Hudson, "Abraham Flexner in Perspective," *Bulletin of the History of Medicine* 46 (November–December 1972): 545–61; and Howard S. Berliner, "A Larger Perspective on the Flexner Report," *International Journal of Health Services* 5:4 (1975): 573–92.

In understanding the significance of Progressive-era medical reform, it is important to keep in mind that nineteenth-century medical practitioners did not enjoy the status and income of the modern-day physician. Relative to other skilled occupational groups, most nineteenth-century doctors felt (and probably were) underpaid and distrusted. It is also important to remember that sectarian competition during this period was fierce. "Regular" or "allopathic" physicians, the ancestors of our contemporary medical establishment, faced challenges from numerous different sects, including homeopaths, eclectics, chiropractors, osteopaths, optometrists, and Christian Scientists.

It should be noted that the pattern of government regulation of the professions bears a marked resemblance to the Progressive "reform" of business, as outlined by Gabriel Kolko, *The Triumph of Conservatism* (Chicago: Quadrangle Books, 1967), and James Weinstein, *The Corporate Ideal in the Liberal State, 1900–1930* (Boston: Beacon Press, 1968).

3. I do not mean to imply by this statement that any licensing law, in and of itself, can produce autonomy and prestige. The history of licensure in eighteenth- and early nineteenth-century America, a period when many states had licensing laws but could not enforce them, effectively disputes this

notion. See Shryock, *Medical Licensing*, esp. chap. 1. The late nineteenth-century laws, which proved much more effective, obviously reflected medicine's new scientific achievements; in other words the change in medicine's legal status reflected the growing efficacy of medical practice. Thus licensing laws have to be viewed in relation to the larger social factors that make them effective or ineffective.

4. The first history of the American registration movement appeared in Adelaide Nutting and Lavinia Dock, *History of Nursing*, 4 vols. (New York: G. P. Putnam and Sons, 1907–12), 3:142–87. Nutting and Dock, two prominent nursing leaders active in the movement themselves, compiled a state-by-state summary of the nurses' legislative efforts. This account still remains the single best history of the registration movement. Subsequent histories have relied heavily on Nutting and Dock, perpetuating its conclusions and biases without adding much further knowledge or interpretation. Two valuable exceptions to this generalization are recent studies of state nurses' associations: Veronica M. Driscoll, *Legitimizing the Profession of Nursing: The Distinct Mission of the New York State Nurses Association* (New York: The Association, 1976); and Carla M. Schissel, "The State Nurses' Association in a Georgia Context," Ph.D. dissertation, Emory University, 1979. This paper owes much to Driscoll's careful legislative history of New York State's successive nurse-practice acts.

5. Lavinia Dock, "What We May Expect from the Law," *American Journal of Nursing* (hereafter cited as *AJN*) 1 (October 1900): 8. I have used published sources in writing this paper, most notably the *Annual Reports* of the New York State Education Department, 1903–20 (hereafter cited as ED–AR). According to ED–8th AR (1912), p. 287, all the papers collected by the examiners prior to 1911 were destroyed in the Capitol Hill fire of that year.

6. These statistics are taken from the U.S. Bureau of the Census, *12th Census* (1900). *Special Reports: Occupation*, p. xxiii. For general overviews of nursing history during this period, see Vern Bullough and Bonnie Bullough, *The Care of the Sick: The Emergence of Modern Nursing* (New York: Prodist, 1978) and Phillip Kalisch and Beatrice Kalisch, *The Advance of American Nursing* (Boston: Little Brown and Co., 1978). Janet James, "Isabel Hampton Robb and the Professionalization of Nursing in the 1890s," in *The Therapeutic Revolution: Essays in the Social History of American Medicine*, ed. by Charles Rosenberg and Morris Vogel (Philadelphia: University of Pennsylvania Press, 1978), pp. 201–44, provides a more detailed perspective on the 1890s, as viewed through the career of one major nursing leader.

7. The concern about overcrowding and lack of standards frequently appeared in appeals for registration. See, for example, Nutting and Dock, *History*, 3:141–43.

8. Annie Goodrich remarked on the New York law in "A General

Presentation of the Statutory Requirements of the Different States," American Society of Superintendents of Training Schools for Nurses, *Proceedings of the 18th Annual Convention*, 1912, p. 218. Charlotte Aikens, "Registration Reports and Some Opinions Concerning Them," *Trained Nurse and Hospital Review* (hereafter cited as *TNHR*) 43 (August 1909): 84.

9. Frank C. Abbott, *Government Policy and Higher Education* (Ithaca: Cornell University Press, 1958), pp. 31–32. (The Regents became part of the Department of Education in 1904.) ED–1st AR (1905), p. 553. John Bardo, "A History of the Legal Regulation of Medical Practice in New York State," *Bulletin of the New York Academy of Medicine* 43 (October 1967): 924–40, remains the only recent account of medical regulation in New York State. ED–4th AR (1908), pp. 342–58, has a useful review of New York's medical practice acts. In 1872 the Regents first received the legal authority to appoint a board of medical examiners with the power to examine and license physicians. Meanwhile the county medical societies and medical colleges still retained the power of licensure they had exercised since the early nineteenth century. In 1880 a law divested the county societies of that power. In 1890 the medical colleges also lost their licensing authority, leaving the Regents the sole source of licensure. The 1890 medical practice act also gave the Regents the power to set preliminary education requirements for medical students and to register all medical schools that met "proper standards." In order to achieve this concentration of power in the Regents, the bill's sponsors had to strike compromises with the "irregular" physicians, who feared sectarian medicine might be discriminated against. Therefore the 1890 act set up three separate medical boards, for regular, eclectic, and homeopathic doctors respectively. The 1907 medical practice act eliminated these separate boards.

10. The text of the nurse registration bill for New York is reprinted in "Official Reports of Societies: New York State Nurses Association," *AJN* 3 (March 1903): 475.

11. As of 1903 nursing and certified public accounting had voluntary registration laws; medicine, law, dentistry, and veterinarian medicine all had mandatory laws. See New York State Department of Education, *Bulletin No. 2*, "The University Law" (1904), for a compilation of the statutes governing the professions. As early as 1900 Sylveen Nye proposed that the nurses' bill protect the term "nurse" by a mandatory law. See Driscoll, *Legitimizing the Profession*, p. 13.

12. The single best primary source for the 1903 debate is "Official Reports of Societies: Report on the New York Bill," 3 (April 1903): 556–62. Driscoll, *Legitimizing the Profession*, pp. 15–18, present a useful recent survey. Susan Armeny, "Resistance to Professionalization by American Trained Nurses, 1890–1905" (Paper presented at the 4th Berkshire Conference, 1978), esp. pp. 15–21, provides an excellent discussion of nursing opposition to the 1903 bill.

13. Champe S. Andrews, "The Campaign for Registration of Nurses in New York State," *AJN* 3 (June 1903): 698, presents the Regent's argument. A. T. Bristow, "What Registration Has Done for the Medical Profession," *AJN* 4 (December 1903): 167, refers to the "hospital men"; Henry R. Hopkins, "Inaugural Address," *Transactions of the Medical Society of the State of New York* (1903), p. 9, calls the trained nurse a "reliable assistant." *The Medical Record, Buffalo Medical Journal,* and *Albany Medical Annals* all had editorials favorable to the 1903 bill. "State Control of Trained Nurses," *AJN* 2 (April 1902): 564. The hospital issue appeared in most discussions of registration's value. "Progress of State Registration: New York," *AJN* 12 (April 1912): 545.

14. The Nurse Board of Examiners devised and administered the registration exam, which was held once a year in several different parts of the state. After marking the exam papers, the examiners published lists of the successful candidates. The inspector of training schools collected reports from the nursing schools, made on-site visits, and determined which institutions met the Regents' minimum standards. The Nurse Advisory Council deliberated on the more sensitive issues involved in setting registration policy, and passed on their recommendations to be approved by the Regents. Of the three types of nurse officials involved in administering the 1903 act, only the inspector had a permanent office in Albany. The examiners and council met periodically to discharge their duties. Annie Goodrich, "Report of the Inspector of Training Schools of New York State," *AJN* 11 (January 1911): 307. Sophia Palmer, "The Effect of Registration Upon the Educational Standards of Training Schools, as Shown by Results in New York State," *AJN* 4 (July 1904): 774.

15. ED–2nd AR (1906), p. 333. Comment by Sophia Palmer on Mary W. McKechnie, "What Has Been Accomplished in the Way of Legislation for Nurses," American Society of Superintendents of Training Schools for Nurses," *Proceedings of the 10th Annual Convention* (1904), p. 66.

16. ED–1st AR (1905), pp. 561–63, outlines the Board of Examiners' first set of requirements.

17. Sophia Palmer, "The Effect of State Registration Upon Training Schools," *AJN* 5 (July 1905): 659, 662. Palmer, "Effect of Registration" (1904), p. 773.

18. Palmer, "The Effect of State Registration" (1905), p. 662. ED–3rd AR (1907), p. 320.

19. Palmer, "Effect of Registration" (1904), p. 774. ED–4th AR (1908), pp. 374–76; ED–5th AR, 3 vols. (1909), 1:362–64. From their development as separate institutions in the early nineteenth century, American mental hospitals had an organizational structure strikingly different from that of the general hospitals. In the asylum one physician had complete charge of the institution, whereas in a general hospital a staff of rotating physicians prevailed. The asylum's "one-man rule" may have made the

mental institution less receptive to the addition of a superintendent of nursing, since she might form a competing source of authority. See Gerald Grob, *Mental Institutions in America* (New York: The Free Press, 1973) for an overview of the asylum's development.

20.   The short quotes are from ED–4th AR (1908), p. 376; ED–5th AR (1909), p. 364. The 1906 syllabus was published as the Department of Education's *Higher Education Bulletin No. 28*. Thereafter the recommended syllabus was revised every few years, to expand on old topics and add new ones, as the content of the registration exam changed. The examiners also published a booklet of rules and information concerning nurse registration, usually referred to as "Handbook No. 13." The handbook carried the list of Regents' approved schools. Annie Goodrich, "Report of the Inspector of Training Schools of New York State," *AJN* 11 (January 1911): 306.

21.   ED–7th AR (1911), 1:220–21. ED–8th AR (1912), pp. 285–86.

22.   ED–8th AR (1912), pp. 285–86. In this report Goodrich graded the state's nursing schools. Of the twenty-two schools she put in the excellent and above average categories, eighteen had bed capacities of over one hundred. Sophia Palmer used the term "regular" schools in "The Effect of Registration" (1904), p. 774. "New York Standards," *AJN* 4 (May 1904): 663.

23.   ED–9th AR (1913), pp. 231–32. Charlotte Aikens, "Preliminary Education and Its Relation to Hospital Problems," *TNHR* 43 (September 1909): 147, noted that the Regents' ruling on this requirement was not being enforced.

24.   ED–9th AR (1913), p. 232.

25.   Ibid., pp. 232–33. A list of hospitals protesting the Regents' ruling can be found in "The Progress of State Registration," p. 543.

26.   Ibid., p. 234.

27.   Augustus Downing, "The New York Nurse Practice Act and Its Administration," *AJN* 12 (December 1911): 190.

28.   The new preliminary education requirement did not have quite the dramatic effect Goodrich and her supporters hoped. Between 1913 and 1917 the number of high school graduates entering the training school, as reported in the ED–ARs, rose from 12 percent to 24 percent; candidates having one or more years of high school from 21 percent to 60 percent. But college-educated women did not enroll in any appreciable numbers until World War I, and the opening of Vassar's Rainbow Camp.

29.   Downing, "The New York Nurse Practice Act," p. 188, states that there were 8,421 R.N.s in 1911. The 1910 census lists 13,862 trained nurses in New York State (U.S. Bureau of the Census, *13th Census Reports*, 11 vols. *Population: Occupation Statistics* 4:124). I have no statistics for R.N.s in 1920, but the census gives 22,935 trained nurses for the state (U.S. Bureau of the Census, *14th Census Reports*, 13 vols. *Population: Occupation Statistics* 4: 984, 986). There were 12,675 trained nurses who registered under the waiver provision of the 1920 act (ED–18th AR [1922], p. 106). These

statistics taken together suggest that the 50-percent figure is fairly accurate, possibly a bit optimistic.

I base these characterizations of the unregistered schools on a comparison of the listings of New York State training schools in United States Bureau of Education, *Annual Report of the Commissioner* (1904) pt. 2, pp. 2162–64; ED–5th AR, 3 vols. (1909), 1:491–94; and ED–16th AR, 3 vols. (1920), 3: 226–30.

30. Goodrich, "Report of the Inspector," p. 306. The number of out-of-state nurses sitting for the registration exam was never reported as a separate figure. Charlotte Aikens, "Registration Reports," p. 88, charged the Education Department with deliberately disguising the low proportion of graduates taking the exam by the misleading way in which the ARs reported these figures. I think her charge may have been justified.

Perhaps the most telling statistic of all reveals that as late as 1920, fully 13 percent of the *superintendents* of approved schools were not R.N.s themselves. This figure can be calculated from tables given in the ED–16th AR, 3 vols. (1920), 3:231–35.

31. See, for example, ED–11th AR, 3 vols. (1915), 1:445, and Annette Fiske, "The Need of Fairness," *TNHR* 51 (July 1913): 6–8. Aikens, "Registration Reports," pp. 86–87.

32. See "Letter to the Editor," *AJN* 5 (January 1905), 158–59; "The Registration Act in New York," ibid., pp. 221–22; and "Registration Deadlock in New York," *TNHR* 34 (June 1905): 370–72. Palmer, "The Effect of Registration" (1904), p. 775. ED–13th AR, 3 vols. (1917), 1:188, states that eleven schools had very high failure rates. Aikens, "Registration Reports," p. 85, states that the state hospital schools were among those with very high numbers of failures.

33. Driscoll, *Legitimizing the Profession*, pp. 23–25. The argument for a mandatory law is nicely stated in Downing, "The New York Nurse Practice Act," and Lucy Ayers, "Future Administration of Registration Laws," *AJN* 13 (September 1913): 957–64.

34. Aikens, "Preliminary Education," p. 152; Aikens, "Registration Reports," p. 85.

35. Driscoll, *Legitimizing the Profession*, pp. 31–32. Charlotte Aikens, "The Registration Movement," *TNHR* 44 (January 1910): 11. See also Driscoll, *Legitimizing the Profession*, pp. 25–32, for a discussion of the opposition's point of view.

36. Ibid., pp. 34–37. The Regents first altered the composition of the Nurse Advisory Council in 1914 in an attempt to help the NYSNA's embattled amendment. Five members representing the state medical society, hospital trustees, and boards of health for the city and state were added to balance the five nurses already on the council. An *AJN* editorial noted that the new council represented both "those in favor of the advance movement and those opposed to it." See "New York Increases Membership of Nurses'

Board of Counsellors," *AJN* 14 (August 1914): 943. Even this change did not satisfy the bill's opponents, who wanted nurses to be a minority on the council.

Almost thirteen thousand nurses registered under the waiver provision of the 1920 nurse practice act (as compared to 5,700 under the 1903 law). Half of those admitted after 1920 were graduates of schools registered by the Regents. ED–18th AR (1922), p. 106.

37.   Driscoll, *Legitimizing the Profession*, p. 35.

38.   Susan Reverby, "The Search for the Hospital Yarkstick," in *Health Care in America*, pp. 206–25.

39.   I do not necessarily share this viewpoint. By examining the nursing leadership's perspective, I by no means wish to imply that the "medical model" of professional uplift they adopted was a wise one. The current problems of the American health care system discourage any such unqualified approval of medicine's professional tactics.

40.   Charlotte Aikens, "Who Should Control in Registration Affairs?" *TNHR* 43 (November 1909): 281. See, for example, Mary Roth Walsh, *Doctors Wanted: No Women Need Apply* (New Haven: Yale University Press, 1977), for a discussion of the negative attitudes toward women doctors.

41.   Veronica Driscoll's analysis makes the connections between the 1903 bill and the landmark Laverne-Pisani bill very explicit. See *Legitimizing the Profession*, esp. pp. 56–73. The New York State registration law for nurses has been amended twice since 1920, in 1938 to require licensing of all who "nurse for hire," and in 1972 to define nursing as distinct from medicine. As Driscoll shows, the same set of conflicting interests that shaped the 1920 act reappeared in these later attempts to amend the licensing law.

7

"Something Besides Waiting": The Politics of Private Duty Nursing Reform in the Depression

Susan Reverby

Those caught in the currents of economic and social upheavals often suffer a very special kind of anguish that comes from a destruction of spirit and hope. Commenting on the "blight of unemployment" for nurses in 1932, Janet Geister, the American Nurses' Association (ANA) director at headquarters, poignantly reminded the delegates to the ANA biennial convention:

> . . . the outstanding evil is not the threat of loss of food and shelter but the destruction of morale that results from the slow, cumulative perception of not being needed. . . . In nursing its destructiveness is proportional to the intensity and universality of the original urge to be of use. But the many nurses who . . . "want work, not charity" are suffering quietly in a way perhaps we will never know.[1]

Six years earlier, Mary Butz, a fifty-year-old, ailing, experienced private duty nurse, wrote not so quietly to Geister of what she called the "*shame*" and "disgrace" of the endless waiting between cases that had come to characterize private duty nursing by the 1920s. The solution to the difficulties lay, she told Geister, in the necessity for "Consideration, Justice, Kindness . . . and to love our neighbors, a little more, not necessarily as much as ourselves." Realizing, however, that more than the Golden Rule and goodwill were necessary, she concluded: "am hoping something besides waiting will be done for nurses waiting for calls."[2]

This "something" was the rapid decline by the end of the depression of the importance of private duty and the simultaneous growth of hospital staff nursing as the major practice field. The explanation by historians for nursing's "great transformation" is usually given as the juncture of several forces: the overproduction and enforced unemployment of nurses and the organized efforts of nursing reformers to introduce graduate staff nursing; the availability of new reimbursement mechanisms for hospital care; the rise of capital-intensive, science- and hospital-based medicine; and shifting morbidity patterns in the society as a whole. Evaluation of this shift from private duty to staff nursing depends on the perspective of the historian. For some, private duty is seen somewhat sentimentally as a way of work sacrificed to the false god of professionalism by the nursing leadership on the altar of rapacious hospitals. For others, its loss is only a measure of the triumph of nursing's long struggle for professional recognition and educational independence.[3]

Despite these differences, historians agree that this change was the inexorable result of economic and social trends intensified by the depression crisis. With the advantage of hindsight, however, these historians tend to see inevitability and not to give enough credence to certain political choices and conflicts made at critical points. In charting the course of this nursing transformation, historians have either ignored or not adequately evaluated an important set of proposed *alternative* reforms that might have eased the human agony of the change and served as counterweights to hospital growth. These reforms sought to find a middle ground between individualized private duty and hospital nursing in the form of what might have become group practices. This article is an examination of an attempt to transform private duty and the pattern of nursing care delivery. While the contours of the contemporary reforms to change the structure of medical care have been outlined, the parallels within nursing have been ignored. Central to the nursing reform efforts, and therefore to this article, were the struggles of ANA director and social reformer Janet Geister as she tried to answer for all nurses Mary Butz's plea that "something besides waiting" had to be done.[4]

Nursing in the 1920s, not unlike a patient with a painful chronic ailment, willingly sought a diagnosis for its ills from its own practitioners and from outside specialists. The numerous opinions confirmed the patient's own suspicions: the problem was both systemic and genetic, inherited from fifty years of dependence and control of its educational program by the hospitals. The ailment took its greatest toll among the majority of nurses to be found in private duty. There were, as one of the diagnoses read, "too many yet too few nurses"—too many without specialized training and good technical and social skills, too few with them.[5]

Medical economist C. Rufus Rorem labeled nursing's problem an "economic paradox" of oversupply and underdemand. "The graduate nurse is in a continuous dilemma," he said in a speech before the National League of Nursing Education (NLNE) convention in 1933. "She cannot find employment as a private duty nurse in the home because more and more patients are going to hospitals. She cannot find employment as a staff nurse in the hospitals because the hospital patients are attended by undergraduate nurses." Further, in the home market she competed, usually unsuccessfully, with the practical and public health nurse. In addition, because of the ambiguousness and low status of home nursing, it became increasingly unpopular with graduate nurses. By the 1920s, therefore, the private duty nurse usually found what employment she could as a "special" for the hospital's private patients.[6]

Private duty was an expensive commodity, which an increasingly smaller percentage of the population could afford to purchase. Never a widely used service, by the late 1920s nearly ten times as many families sought medical care as they did private duty nursing. Income rather than medical or nursing need determined the demand: 9 percent of the population with incomes over $5,000 a year received more than half the private duty nursing services. In addition private duty care was still bought in increments of twelve to twenty-four hours, so that it often represented a larger purchase than either physicians' services or hospital care. Private duty nurses were working primarily for the well-to-do, either solving their "servant problem" in the home or, by acting as specials, shoring up and perpetuating the hospital's inadequate student nursing service.[7]

The decline in the amount of sickness that constituted the "bread-and-butter" illnesses for the private duty nurse further aggravated the employment situation. As Janet Geister noted, "gone were the weeks the private duty nurse spent caring for victims of typhoid, pneumonia, la grippe, yellow fever, malaria and intestinal diseases." The expanding hospital surgical and maternity services, and the growing public acceptance of hospital-based care, transferred the appendectomy patient from the kitchen table to an operating theater and the parturient woman from the bedroom to a delivery suite. Frances Ott, a leader of the Private Duty Nursing section of the ANA, reminisced in 1932:

Time was when all you had to say was you were a nurse and you wanted something to do and the first thing you knew you had a case. . . . I know when I went to Chicago in 1892 I spent one day getting a room, one day in looking around and the next day I had a typhoid fever case for the next three weeks. I made more in that year than I could now in five or six years.

This was not just another depression story. By 1926 the average private duty nurse in New York was out of work over four months of the year. Yet ironically, the Committee on the Costs of Medical Care studies indicated nonhospital-based nursing met only 40 percent of the community nursing needs.[8]

The irrational distribution system of private duty nursing further complicated the situation. As private, individual workers, the private duty nurse found her cases through word of mouth; city directory listings; referrals from physicians, patients, or druggists; and nursing registries. Registries were run by medical and nursing societies, hospitals and commercial interests. In any given city any number of registries could exist with differing standards, prices, and available services. Because the system did not grade the graduate nurses, nursing charges were set by the registry and did not vary with experience. As nurses' complaints about the unfairness of the registries began to be vocalized in the 1890s, some of the leaders in nursing sought to gain nursing control over their operations and to discuss the necessity for making them both more democratic and more responsive to community needs. By the 1910s the ANA began to promote the organization of registries that were centralized and officially sponsored by nursing organizations; but by 1926 only half the registries in the country were conducted by central nursing organizations and it was often impossible to distinguish commercial ventures from nursing ones.[9]

Hospital and alumnae registries were frequently very small and supplied only their own graduates as specials in their hospitals. The commercial agencies, which received a percentage on each case, thus profited by supplying some kind of nurse, either graduate or practical, and were often better able to meet the broader and varied demands for nursing services in the community. In Boston the commercially run Beal Nurses' Home and Registry, Inc. had an hourly nursing service as early as 1913 and advertised that "doctors practicing among the salaried classes are particularly enthusiastic about it." At a turbulent discussion at the ANA convention in 1924, for example, nurses admitted that the commercial agencies often allowed the more experienced graduate nurses to charge more, thus making them more attractive than the official nursing registries. Thus the registries at best functioned only as nursing employment agencies or hiring halls for hospital specials, rather than as either community services or professional organizations. They were the continual focus of nursing discontent and concern.[10]

As with all economic paradoxes, the nursing situation posed a concomitant political and social difficulty. Those who stayed in private duty, the majority of whom were graduates of the smaller nursing schools, were often less educated and less prepared than nurses in either institutional or public health positions. When they worked they were sequestered in patients' homes or private hospital rooms for 84 to 168 hours a week. When they weren't working, they were waiting at home for calls. This left little time for outside interests, organized activities, or nursing politics. In private duty there was no organized professional growth, no supervision, no certainty. "Her life isolates her from society," Janet Geister wrote sympathetically in her report on private duty in 1926:

> . . . its irregularity breaks down her health, its seclusions tend to narrow her interests. She cannot charge in accordance with any particular skill she has acquired; she is unethical if, after ten years of hard work, she charges any more than does the newest graduate in the field. Yet she must be all things to all people, she must remain human though she cannot live like most humans.[11]

By the mid-1920s such women had grown increasingly bitter over their unemployment and defensive about their lack of education and skills. A New York private duty nurse wrote: "I intend to keep on doing private nursing because I don't know anything else; wish I never had to see another patient again." The freedom to give total bedside care, to work when she wanted, and to be independent of the yoke of hospital supervision was purchased at the expense of low income, lack of rest, constant worry, and the nagging sense that she was seen by the patients, doctors, and other nurses as a "menial servant" doing "lady's-maid" work. As the private duty nurse aged, the allure of youthful independence gave way to the difficult realities of increasing unemployment. "I am forty-eight years of age and have the best of health," a Washington private duty nurse stated. "I feel quite peppy, but I can see this is the age of youth, and I want to give up nursing before I get to be a tired old nurse that people pity." Over half the private duty nurses queried by nursing's Grading Committee reported they would leave private duty if they could. But not so the older and less educated women for whom there was no place to go. "Have not been able to save enough money to do otherwise," another New York nurse wrote, "and am untrained for any other kind of work and now am too old to train."[12]

This discontent, although widespread, was not yet organized. A private duty nursing section of the ANA was formed in 1916, but it played very little role in the association's ongoing life and only really met at the conventions. In 1919 Massachusetts claimed to have the only thoroughly well-organized Private Duty League; it had eighty-one members. Specific coalitions on the local level were formed, particularly around legislative issues, but did not and could not sustain their efforts.[13]

Nor did private duty nurses have a real spokeswoman to voice their concerns and focus their demands. Annette Fiske, a graduate of the Waltham Training School with an advanced degree from Radcliffe, spoke out articulately at many nursing meetings and wrote numerous articles in support of the private duty nurse. She placed the blame for the difficulties in nursing on the "training schools and nursing leadership, not on individual nurses or hospitals or physicians." But her solutions to the problems only emphasized the necessity for valuing the nurse's "spirit of service" and her "most skillful and kindly care of the sick." The *Trained Nurse* journal, in which her views appeared, took a similar position in its support for private duty nurses and its attacks on the educational reform strategies of the nursing leadership. But the dilemmas of the 1920s called for a political language and effort that spoke to self-renewal and organizations, not self-abnegation and individual effort.[14]

The political language of the nursing leadership by the 1920s focused on the facts of the present and their consequences for nursing, and did not offer hosannas to some lost nursing past. The Grading Committee studies, financed by foundation funds, nursing benefactors, and thousands of individual nurses, were one of the key efforts to analyze the nursing dilemma and make recommendations for change. These studies in particular quantified the arguments of a generation of nursing leaders that the private duty nursing problem was caused by overproduction and low standards. Their solution focused on calls to cut off the production of nursing students, to raise educational standards, to separate the nursing service from nursing education by placing hospital nursing in the hands of graduates.[15]

Despite this response to the crisis, there was very little real concern for the dilemmas of the individual private duty nurse. The leadership appeared to share the aphorism repeated in a Grading Committee study that "every nurse ought to do some private duty, but no good nurse ought to stay in the field more than a few years." Most nursing leaders appeared to follow this dictum in their career patterns and they were almost all public health nurses, educators, or superintendents. Authority and private duty nursing were considered contradictory principles. The typical biographical sketch of a nurse with any official authority read repeatedly, "after a period of private duty she became superintendent of nurses, or a public health nursing leader." But the leadership was also well aware that the public's and the physician's perception of nursing were shaped more by their encounters with the individual nurse than with the pronouncements from nursing headquarters or the career patterns of the more successful few.[16]

The leadership perceived the crisis as primarily a serious dilemma for nursing's professional status and its educational goals. In December 1928, for example, Teachers College nursing professor Elizabeth Burgess wrote to the director of the Grading Committee, May Ayers Burgess (no relation), to ask her opinion on what ought to be done in light of the Grading Committee's factual findings. May Ayers Burgess answered that the nursing leadership was "faced with a bald set of facts which are rather dreadful to think about." After listing the data on oversupply and undereducation of nursing graduates she added:

> Dissatisfaction and unrest are particularly noticeable in what might be called the non-professional nursing ranks. The expressions of this unrest are not always fortunate. Out of every ten active graduate nurses in the United States, three belong to the ANA, seven do not. Control of the nursing profession now rests in the hands of a small minority body.

She concluded: "the events of the next two or three years may perhaps determine whether nursing is to be a real profession or whether it is to be one of what the U.S. Census calls the 'Domestic and Personal Service Occupation.'"[17]

May Ayers Burgess and others in nursing saw the problem in class terms. Burgess publicly stated that since many nurses were drawn from families "not strictly professional in character" they were making "trouble within the profession." Trouble and unfortunate expressions of "unrest" were her words for the beginnings of open discussions of unions. These women, she declared:

> are less and less inclined to accept leadership from other nurses whose academic and social backgrounds are better, and they are increasingly inclined to stand apart and work bitterly for what seems to them the only possible economic solution for their difficulties. The worse unemployment becomes, the more difficulty the profession will inevitably face in handling this group of its members.

"Fortunately," she concluded, "there is no longer any need for them."[18] In the interim "such women" were the majority in nursing and some way had to be devised to quiet their discontent and meet their needs. One solution appears to have been the ANA Board of Directors' offer in 1926 of the position as director at headquarters to nurse and social reformer Janet Geister.

Geister was in an excellent position to become the spokeswoman for the private duty nurse. She had just completed and presented at the May 1926 ANA convention a major well-acclaimed study entitled "Hearsay and Facts in Private Duty." Coming two years before the publication of the Grading Committee's study *Nurses, Patients and Pocketbooks*, Geister's report was the first sympathetic factual discussion of the private duty nursing problem. Clearly tapping into a well of unmet needs, she was immediately besieged by requests from over half a dozen state nursing associations to speak on the issues. But, she wrote to the ANA president, S. Lillian Clayton, it was impossible for her to leave her current job to fulfill the requests. She asked Clayton if the ANA or the Grading Committee, more appropriately, could take on this work. A month after she wrote Clayton she was informally queried as to her interest in the position as the ANA's Director of Headquarters. Three months later, in October 1926, the ANA Board unanimously offered her the job.[19]

Janet Geister was perhaps a perfect and seemingly safe choice for the position. A 1910 graduate of a small hospital training school outside Chicago, she spent a year in private duty. "It didn't satisfy me," she wrote in unpublished biographical notes, "I wanted to get at *causes*." In this quest she enrolled at the Chicago School of Civics and Philanthropy and received her theoretical education as a social reformer under the tutelage of Jane Addams, Julia Lathrop, Graham Taylor, and Alice Hamilton. Rather than accept a number of executive positions offered upon completion of this training, she chose to experience life in the field. She spent several years as an infant welfare nurse, a medical social worker, and a supervisor in the Chicago Visiting Nurse Association. Julia Lathrop lured her away to the Children's Bureau in 1917 to do field research on infant and maternal mortality and day-care facilities. In the early 1920s she became the field and then educational secretary of the National Organization of Public Health Nursing (NOPHN) and a researcher for the Cleveland Hospitals and Health Survey, the Goldmark Report, and a survey of public health nursing. Most of her fieldwork brought her in daily contact with the concerns of working nurses and fostered her respect for their efforts. "I . . . came to believe," she recalled, "that there is no finer way to appraise a nurse than to walk with her and talk with her as she works. . . . Everywhere too, I found nurses quietly performing miracles in improving the health life of families."[20]

Medical reformer Michael Davis hired her in 1923 to be part of his interdisciplinary staff on a major study of the New York City dispensaries. In the rich intellectual atmosphere of this project, Geister was exposed to the positive aspects of molding diverse and strongly held opinions into a common purpose and to the use of fact-finding to set standards and to make changes in actual practice. While on the project staff she organized the independent study that became "Hearsay and Facts." Thus Geister brought to the ANA respect for the working nurse, no real loyalties to any nursing organization except perhaps the NOPHN, and a commitment, as she described it, to "cold appraisals and strong action." She was part of a group of health reformers who had, in the words of one of her contemporaries, "a deep-seated confidence that concerted study, analysis and reflection on the part of knowledgeable and concerned people could result in a program useful for dealing with problems that called for societal resolution.[21]

The problem that captured her imagination and concern was that of the private duty nurse. Writing to the *Trained Nurse*'s editor in 1941, she requested: "when and if you write my obituary this is the one thing I'd like emphasized—that I wanted to get down to brass tacks for the private duty nurse." She agreed that the private duty nurse was "ill-adjusted and poorly trained" but, unlike May Ayers Burgess, she saw this as a challenge, not a burden for nursing. In 1928, just a month before Burgess wrote about the danger of unrest, Geister reported to the ANA's Board of Directors on her field trip to attend nursing meetings in eight states. She commented on the unemployment and "greater despair in the private duty ranks." She too was fearful about how this unrest would be expressed. But in contrast to Burgess she perceived a "willingness and eagerness" on the part of these women to accept the national's leadership, signified by their overwhelming personal financial support of the costs of the Grading Committee's work and their openness to her.[22]

Geister wanted nursing to face squarely the realities of the social and structural shifts of the twentieth century. She saw the nation's nursing needs for the ever increasing care of the chronic and convalescent patient. "The collective production of medicine," she believed, was clearly the "wave of the future." She wanted nurses to understand this and to shape their own future, not mourn their past. She worried that the private duty nurse, if left alone, would become increasingly bitter and estranged, while nursing would be continually criticized for not meeting the public's needs. Teamwork and the necessity for what she called the "radical reorganization of the private duty nursing system" appeared obvious. She cited the demise of the teacher tutoring an individual pupil and the shoemaker creating a shoe by hand as analogous to the private duty situation. Collective and machine-aided work, she declared, made their commodities available to a broader range of consumers and increased the demand for workers. She claimed that a parallel shift was both inevitable and positive for nursing.[23]

Above all Geister saw the necessity for action; and action meant the acceptance of conflict. She thought a willingness to question those in authority and to tackle controversies were signs not of disloyalty, but of growth. Uncertainty and social experimentation were to be valued not feared. Atrophy and inertia were the sins; change and conflict were not. Geister believed, however, in guided evolution, not revolution. The transformation of nursing had to be managed by those in responsible leadership.[24]

The ANA, as nursing's major organization, had the responsibility, she believed, actively to assist their rank and file to make this shift to the modern world. Something "drastic," she argued, had to be done "for those who are already in the field and who will be there for years to come. We may set up our ideals and hopes but for a long time we shall be faced with the practical facts of the enormously uneven quality in service of nurses. . . . How shall the salvaging and leveling off be done?" She did not disagree with the nursing reformers' hopes that changes had to be made at the point of production of *trained nurses*. But she earnestly directed her energies toward the point of production of *nursing care*, which was in part the distribution system. Her fieldwork and contacts gave her the sense that support and concern existed in the nursing and wider communities for such a strategy. Well aware of the work of the Committee on the Costs of Medical Care, for example, she wanted nursing to keep up with the new currents in the health delivery system.[25]

Her strategic sense led her to focus her concern with distribution on the nursing registry as "the greatest single agency available for the solution of the private duty nurse's problem." Geister had a vision not of the registry as it was, but of what it might become. Expanding on recommendations expressed in the Goldmark and Grading Committee reports, she wanted it transformed into something akin to a nursing group practice. The reorganized registry would have an appointment schedule, varieties of services available, graded and supervised work, and an administrative structure not unlike that of the visiting nurse associations (VNAs). She saw it as a "cooperative venture," which would become a nursing service bureau to meet the community's and nursing's needs. As the central distributing station for nursing, it could institute "need-based" planning and shape its services to meet those needs. It would also educate the public as to the potential uses of nursing in a more professional, less demeaning manner and on a more limited time basis. With a graded service the worry over the role for practical nurses could be lessened. In cooperation with the VNAs, she saw the registry as revitalizing a role for graduate nurses outside the hospital's walls. For the nurse, and even the nursing student, the registry (rechristened a nursing bureau) would become a "teaching and promotion center." It would be a place for the nurse to receive supervision and gain in nursing skills. It could be a mechanism through which to reach the isolated and unorganized private duty nurse "to guide her into the new adjustments in practice and help her find new fields of work."[26]

She was aware of the difficulties of the transformation she was proposing and of the problems of helping nurses actively to "translate facts into actions." She knew that the reorganized registry could be perceived as a threat, in particular, to public health nursing interests, who were at the time experimenting with hourly nursing and the expansion of the social class base of their clientele. She spoke over and over again about the necessity for "cooperation in nursing" and the eventual control of the registry by representatives from all of nursing, medicine, and the public. But such change had to come in increments.[27]

Incremental change, however, did not mean inaction. Geister actively supported the introduction of hospital staff nursing as well, but she saw the wider need for nursing services in the community. Her immediate tactical plan was to use the ANA's rather dormant Committee on Registries to provide minimal standards and concrete assistance on the local level. Under her tutelage the committee geared up and began to send out questionnaires, tabulate facts, and set standards, but always, as Geister stated, as a way to "stimulate thinking and to provide a practical advisory field service to aid local planning." She consistently urged the ANA Board of Directors to sponsor more local institutes and regional, state, and divisional conferences, to begin a larger advisory service at Headquarters, and to seek foundation support for nursing service experiments in various communities. Assessing the ANA's budget, she wanted a shift in priorities toward more spending on service for the local levels and less on structures and the dues for the International Council of Nurses. At a time when the nation's nursing system was clearly in disarray and transition, she attempted to commit the energies of nursing's largest and strongest association to concrete plans to rebuild a viable and more broadly based, organized nursing system.[28]

Such a service program necessitated that organized nursing reorient itself from self-assessment to self-action. It demanded that the masses of facts and recommendations be translated into strategies for change. The open conflict that Geister thought necessary became instead closed personal and organizational infighting. Her six years at the ANA were characterized by growing tensions between her and the women close to the ANA's president, Elnora Thomson, and Geister's increasing inability to have her proposals seriously considered. Personalities and the inherent structural tensions between an organization's board and its staff played a significant role in her difficulties. From all reports Geister was a somewhat unsophisticated figure, given to handing out rabbits' feet to friends, unable or unwilling to meet the ladylike public standards of nursing behavior, and not well versed in organizational infighting. Furthermore, the paramilitary and parareligious nursing culture demanded personal and organizational loyalty and obedience as its first law, but unquestioning fealty was inimical to Geister's character. In January 1933 Geister was finally rather summarily forced to resign her position by the ANA Board. The private duty nurse was left to founder without, as a Geister supporter lamented, "their understanding Friend" at headquarters.[29]

A difference over what kind of reform effort there should be in nursing, a reliance on symbolic politics, and the threat to public health nursing of her proposals all suffused the conflict. Much more than a personality conflict was in question here. For forty years, nursing leaders had concentrated their efforts on nursing education and the system of producing student nurses. They placed their hopes on gaining support for a Flexner-type reform, which would have closed the weaker schools and upgraded nursing educational requirements and programs. Geister's strategy would have forced them to confront the question of distribution and to accept the necessity for upgrading those already in the profession.

Such problems could hardly be ignored. Beginning in 1928 the ANA did heavily finance a Joint Committee on Distribution with the NLNE and NOPHN. It had twenty-four members, none of whom was a private duty nurse, a complicated subcommittee structure responsible for almost every major distributional issue in nursing (including the introduction of staff nursing), and a secretary who was committed to office research rather than field studies. In January 1932, the year before Geister was dismissed, the ANA president engineered a bureaucratic maneuver to have the independent Registry Committee become a subcommittee of the Distribution Committee, thereby effectively burying the registry work. The chairwoman of the Distribution Committee at the time, who was the director of Buffalo's VNA, reportedly told her committee's secretary, "We will just let the registry matters go for awhile. The registry has had plenty of attention." For more than three years, at the zenith of private duty unemployment, the registry work was tabled and only minor revisions in the Registry Committee's standards were made.[30]

Geister's rhetoric about community nursing services was adopted, but not the office and local support necessary for real implementation. In 1934 the Distribution Committee considered its work done and dissolved, and yet another ANA Registry Committee organized. It lasted a year and then headquarters staff took over all its work along with their other responsibilities. On the surface all the right things were done: they too sent out questionnaires, tabulated monthly registry reports, conducted some field surveys, and discussed the community service idea, but energetic commitment to transforming private duty and to assisting the private duty nurse was not made. Although some placement service work was done, the results were mainly used to focus curriculum planning. By the closing years of the 1930s, with the growth of Blue Cross financing for hospital care and the increasing employment of nurses in staff positions, this was too little too late. At midcentury, nursing leader Mary Roberts, never a Geister supporter, could write of the registries: "the scope of their services and methods of integrating them with other professional services were still not clearly defined." Twenty years later nursing historian Teresa Christy would echo this sentiment.[31]

The problems of the private duty nurse and the necessity for matching community needs to nursing resources were not directly addressed. In 1934 still another joint committee was authorized, this time on Community Nursing Service. Led by public health nurses and educators, it looked into community nursing needs and encouraged the formation of community nursing councils. It spent years determining its priorities and preparing a survey instrument and standards, and also did some field work. Alma Haupt, a prominent public health nurse on the committee, commented during a particularly difficult bureaucratic wrangle in 1938: "Couldn't we agree from past and present experience that a joint committee such as this one is necessary, if for nothing more than to serve as a symbol of the unity of the three national organizations?"[32]

Fact-finding and standard-making, without an increasing commitment to ongoing field surveys and continued encouragement of local efforts, did remain primarily a symbol of organizational rather than membership unity. But as Geister had argued, service and experimentation, not symbolic politics, were necessary to solve the nursing dilemma. In 1939 medical reformer Michael Davis issued a challenge to professional nursing by politely congratulating them for the "consciousness" of knowing there was a necessity to measure and match nursing needs to services. But, he pointedly declared, such a consciousness "had not been taken seriously in a practically effective way."[33]

Finally, Geister's ideas were never really tested because they were perceived to be in conflict with the interests of public health nursing. She denied that the reorganized and strengthened registry had to be a threat to the public health field. "There was ample room for both," she thought. But others in more powerful positions in nursing did not believe such sharing was possible. She alleged that her final programmatic suggestions for the ANA were labeled "dangerous" by a public health nursing administrator on the ANA Board of Directors and that the organization's president remarked: "You would have the ANA mixed up with community activities. We refer these things to the NOPHN."[34]

After much debate within public health nursing in the 1920s, a consensus was developing that this practice field would provide generalized nursing care, both preventive and curative, for the entire community. This included, along with the traditional charitable visit, the offering of a partial fee system and an hourly or appointment service with fees to attract the patient of "moderate means." Further, the voluntary, or nonofficial, agencies faced an increasing fiscal crisis in the 1920s and the early 1930s as the demand for their services threatened constantly to outstrip their charitable income. There was thus both an ideological and a financial aspect to their hopes that broadening the appeal and services of public health nursing agencies would allow them to become more than a charity.[35]

Geister believed that public health nursing was too identified in the public mind with a charity service and too preoccupied with its other services ever to put enough effort into this kind of expansion. She never opposed the VNAs providing hourly services, however. She was arguing for experimentation in structure, not the closing off of possibilities due to narrow interests. She also doubted that a field enormously concerned with raising the educational standards and the preparation of its practitioners would be willing to be flooded by ill-prepared women. In her final program report to the ANA in 1932 she applauded the efficiency and high standards of work of the VNAs, but asked rhetorically: "Is the VNA prepared to take over the professional problems that now perplex the well conducted registry—vocational guidance, grading the service etc. as well as to act as a general distributing center for all types of nurses in the community?"[36]

Indeed the VNAs decreased in number as the official, or governmentally sponsored, public health agencies increased in number and size.

These agencies, which provided primarily preventive services for the poor, undermined the vision of public health nursing as a broad community service and further linked it with charity services. In addition the development of community-chest funding in some cities for the voluntary agencies, and their fear of alienating their charitable contributors, blunted the VNAs' urgency on experimenting with new service modes. An examination of VNA annual reports and the statistics of the NOPHN led Michael Davis to conclude in 1939 that the agencies' attempts to provide hourly services had been half-hearted and would not work "until it and the work of the visiting nurse association in general are closely related to the local registry for private duty nurses."[37]

Although forced out of the ANA, Geister did not give up easily. Her dismissal caused a mild furor all over the country in a variety of nursing circles, but many of her supporters were not privy to the details of headquarters' fights. She explained the circumstances and politics of her situation to a select few. Clearly physically and emotionally exhausted by six years of conflict and more concerned with nursing's growth than her career, she squelched a movement to demand her reinstatement. On a strong platform that reflected her ideas, she ran as part of an oppositional slate for secretary of the ANA in 1934. But the power of the entrenched officers and, she alleged, some last-minute political manipulations cost her this election.[38]

Geister's concerns did not dissolve along with her position. She became an editor of the *Trained Nurse* and continued to support the needs of both private duty and staff nurses through her voluminous writings and nursing activism. After the war, in fact, she was elected to the ANA Board. In 1935 she wrote that "if nursing continues its laissez-faire policy on the matter of adequate distribution and continues to work on production, we're going to find ourselves in an even worse jam in a few years." Twenty-eight years later, in 1963, the year before her death, she wrote: "time has not changed my belief these programs were needed. Private duty has not died, but the aimless drifting of today's private practice and its miscellaneous quality is not good." The focus on education reforms, she declared, left nursing with its "present hospital nursing problems" because of the lack of as much concern with "administrative practices" and "employment conditions." But more importantly, she worried then, as she always did, about the damage to the *spirit* within nursing, rather than its structures.[39]

Even if her programmatic suggestions had been carried out, they might not have been able to stave off the social and economic forces that underlay the development of hospital-based care. Previous attempts by other groups of workers to form the kinds of cooperatives she proposed did not often last in the face of the power of industrial capital. Similarly the more powerful reformers with compatible views to hers on the Committee on the Costs of Medical Care lost out to the entrenched forces of the American Medical Association. The committee may have created the ideological climate that made possible the beginning growth of prepaid group practices in medicine, but they too were unable to implement the broad structural reforms they sought. Nor perhaps could the financing have been found at that time to pay for such ambulatory nursing care, except in a few foundation-supported settings or small communities. Nor is it clear that nurses or the public would have easily accepted the reforms she advocated. In 1936, for example, when the Waltham Training School for Nurses in Waltham, Massachusetts, closed, the school's trustees set up a nursing service bureau for the community. The bureau sent out almost half its nurses on hourly nursing calls, but reported that the public mainly demanded attendants or mother's helpers. Nor finally is it certain her strategy could have healed the divisions within nursing or given nurses the "something besides waiting" that they needed.[40]

Geister tapped into the discontent of nursing's rank and file and articulated their concerns. The question of whether her solutions would have worked is less relevant than our understanding the importance of her willingness to offer more than pity or disdain to the women trapped by the nursing system. Her ideas were never given a real chance for implementation and their potential never really tested. Her program was too much of a threat to both nursing's reform efforts and its cultural style. As historians, however, we have a responsibility to explain what *did not* happen in nursing as well as to chronicle what *did*.

NOTES

The research for this paper was done under Grant No. 1 RO3 HS 02879–01 from the National Center for Health Services Research, DHSS. I wish to thank Janet Golden, Diana Long Hall, Ellen Lagemann, Eric Schneider, Tim Sieber, and Nancy Tomes for their comments on an earlier draft. I am more than grateful to Karen Buhler-Wilkerson for sharing her work and her understanding of the nursing culture with me. Grateful acknowledgment is made to Dorothy Weber and Boston University for use of the Janet Geister Papers and to Teachers College for use of the Isabel M. Stewart Papers.

1. "Report of the Director at Headquarters to House of Delegates, January 1932," Janet Geister Papers, Box 10, Folder 89, Nursing Archives, Mugar Library, Special Collections, Boston University, Boston, Mass.

2. Mary Butz to Janet Geister (hereafter cited as JG), Nov. 24, 1926, Box 14, Folder 113, Geister Papers.

3. See, for examples of the usual historical explanations, Mary Roberts, *American Nursing: History and Interpretation* (New York: Macmillan, 1954); Philip A. Kalisch and Beatrice J. Kalisch, *The Advance of American Nursing* (Boston: Little, Brown and Co., 1978); Kathleen Cannings and William Lazonick, "The Development of the Nursing Labor Force in the United States: A Basic Analysis," *International Journal of Health Services* 5:2 (1975): 185–217; David Wagner, "The Proletarianization of Nursing in the United States, 1932–1946," ibid. 10:2 (1980): 271–90. I would also include in this viewpoint my earlier, "The Search for the Hospital Yardstick: Nursing and the Rationalization of Hospital Work," in *Health Care in America: Essays in Social History*, ed. Susan Reverby and David Rosner (Philadelphia: Temple University Press, 1979), pp. 206–25, and "Re-forming the Hospital Nurse: The Management of American Nursing," in *The Sociology of Health and Illness, Critical Perspectives*, ed. Peter Conrad and Rochelle Kern (New York: St. Martin's Press, 1981), pp. 220–32.

On private duty see, in particular, Wagner, "The Proletarianization of Nursing," pp. 272–75. For a different view on the ambiguities of private duty, see Susan Reverby, "'Neither for the Drawing Room nor for the Kitchen': Private Duty Nursing in Boston, 1880–1912" (Paper presented at the Organization of American Historians Annual Meeting, April 15, 1978). For the professional triumph view, see Roberts, *American Nursing*, pp. 162–327; Kalisch and Kalisch, *The Advance of American Nursing*, pp. 327–444.

4. Geister has remained invisible in nursing histories. Her role is not discussed in any of the major histories, although her articles on private duty and staff nursing are cited both by Kalisch and Kalisch and by Wagner. The work of the ANA's directors is not discussed in *One Strong Voice: The Story of the American Nurses' Association*, compiled by Lyndia Flanagan (Kansas City: American Nurses' Association, 1976). The only rather cryptic hints on the conflict surrounding Geister can be found in Stella Goostray, *Memoirs: Half a Century in Nursing* (Boston: Nursing Archive, 1969), p. 67. Professor Virginia Deforge of the Boston University School of Nursing is now beginning a full-scale biography of Geister.

Geister's printed writings, her papers, and the papers of the American Nurses' Association, all in the Nursing Archives at Boston University, can be used to recreate the conflicts.

5. Josephine Goldmark, *Nursing and Nursing Education in the United States. Report of the Committee for the Study of Nursing Education and a Report of a Survey by Josephine Goldmark* (New York: Macmillan, 1923); Committee on the Grading of Nursing Schools, *Nurses, Patients and Pocketbooks* (New York: The Committee, 1928); The Committee, *Nurses: Production, Education, Distribution, and Pay* (New York: The Committee, 1930); The Committee, *Results of the First Grading Study of Nursing*

Schools, 3 vols. (New York: National League of Nursing Education, 1931); National Organization of Public Health Nursing, *Report of the Committee to Study Visiting Nursing* (New York: The Organization, 1924); Committee on the Grading of Nursing Schools, Final Report, *Nursing Schools, Today and Tomorrow* (New York: The Committee, 1934), pp. 22–60.

6. "Nursing—An Economic Paradox," *Proceedings 39th Annual Convention, National League of Nursing Education, 1933* (New York: NLNE, 1933), p. 119. On private duty employment see, Grading Committee, *Nurses, Patients and Pocketbooks*, pp. 66–86, 96–98; "The Registry Looks at the Private Duty Nurse," *American Journal of Nursing* (hereafter cited as *AJN*) 29 (December 1929): 1465; Roberts, *American Nursing*, pp. 117–24. The records of individual registries can be used somewhat as a guide to this change toward hospital specialing; see, for example, *Annual Reports of the Suffolk County Nurses Central Directory*, District Five Massachusetts State Nurses Association Papers, Box 1, Nursing Archives. However, because individual registries often specialized themselves in one type of service, these kinds of records are not a good guide to overall shifts, nor can the shift from home-based to hospital-based private duty be accurately dated.

7. Rorem, "Nursing—An Economic Paradox," pp. 115–16. Rorem was citing data later published in I. S. Falk, C. Rufus Rorem, Martha D. Ring, *The Costs of Medical Care* (Chicago: University of Chicago Press, 1933). The purchase of private duty nursing by primarily the well-to-do was not a new phenomenon; see Reverby, " 'Neither for the Kitchen nor for the Drawing Room.' " See also Grading Committee, *Nurses, Patients and Pocketbooks*, pp. 317–61; JG, "Hearsay and Facts in Private Duty," *AJN* 26 (July 1926): 520.

8. JG, "Private Duty Nursing Then—And Now," *Trained Nurse and Hospital Review* (hereafter cited as *TNHR*) 100 (April 1938): 383–86, 445; Frances Ott speech in *Proceedings of the 28th Convention (April 10–15, 1932) of the American Nurses' Association* (New York: American Nurses' Association, 1932), p. 201; JG, "Hearsay and Facts in Private Duty," p. 521; I. S. Falk, Margaret C. Klem, and Nathan Sinai, *The Incidence of Illness and the Receipt and Costs of Medical Care Among Representative Families* (Chicago: University of Chicago Press, 1933), p. 288; Roger I. Lee and Lewis Webster Jones, *The Fundamentals of Good Medical Care* (Chicago: University of Chicago Press, 1933), pp. 121–25; Michael M. Davis, "Nursing Service Measured by Social Needs," *AJN* 39 (January 1939): 35–43.

9. See Roberts, *American Nursing*, 117–24; Lavinia L. Dock, "Directories for Nurses," *First and Second Annual Reports of the American Society of Superintendents of Training Schools for Nurses, 1895*, pp. 56–60; Dock, "Training Schools and Registries," *TNHR* 21 (August 1898); 65–68; Louise Darche, "Proper Organization of Training Schools in America," *Nursing of the Sick, 1893* (New York: McGraw-Hill, 1949), pp. 93–106; JG, "Pri-

vate Duty Nursing Then—and Now"; Reverby, " 'Neither for the Drawing Room nor for the Kitchen' "; Grading Committee, *Nurses, Patients and Pocketbooks*, p. 86. See, for example, Ella Best, "The Rhode Island State Nurses Association Report of Registry Study with Community Implications," ANA Board of Directors Minutes, Jan. 23–25, 1935 Exhibit V(a), ANA Papers, Box 42, Nursing Archives.

10.   The Beal agency used only graduate nurses and later became part of the Suffolk County Nurses Central Directory. "Hourly Nursing in Boston," *TNHR* 50 (January 1913): 40–41, and advertisement in *TNHR* 50 (February 1913): 112; "Private Duty Problems," *TNHR* 73 (July 1924): 57–58. For a similar viewpoint of the difficulties with official vs. commercial registries, see Roberts, *American Nursing*, pp. 117–24.

11.   Grading Committee, *Nurses, Patients and Pocketbooks*, pp. 251–57. Of the nurses in public health 88 percent had done some private duty, and 74 percent of the nurses in staff nursing had. JG, "Hearsay and Facts in Private Duty," p. 518.

12.   Grading Committee, *Nurses, Patients and Pocketbooks*, pp. 311–14, 359–60, 363, 388.

13.   Flanagan, *One Strong Voice*, passim; *Proceedings First Annual Convention of New England Nurses, June 1919*, Massachusetts Nurses Association Papers, Box 7, Nursing Archives; Susan Armeny, "Resistance to Professionalization by American Trained Nurses, 1890–1905" (Paper presented at the Berkshire Conference on the History of Women, Aug. 25, 1978).

14.   See, for example, Annette Fiske, "Nursing—As a Profession Where to Place the Emphasis, *TNHR* 72 (March 1924): 227–28; "Has the Nursing Instinct Died Out? A Plea for a Genuineness of Purpose," *TNHR* 73 (November 1924): 438–39; "The Future of the Private Duty Nurse," *Proceedings First Annual Convention of New England Nurses*, p. 48; "Nursing as a Profession," *The Radcliffe Magazine* 16 (February 1914): 92–95. For a further discussion of Fiske's role, see Susan Reverby, "The Nursing Disorder: A Critical History of the Hospital-Nursing Relationship, 1860–1945" (Ph.D. dissertation, Boston University, 1982). I am grateful to Jane Knowles of the Schlesinger Library at Radcliffe College for making Fiske's student records available. The *TNHR* was the main oppositional journal in nursing from the 1880s until it folded in 1957. On the importance of the language of politics, see J. G. A. Pocock, *Politics, Language and Time: Essays on Political Thought and History* (New York: Atheneum, 1971).

15.   M. Adelaide Nutting, *Sound Economic Basis for Schools of Nursing and Other Addresses* (New York: G. P. Putnam's Sons, 1926); Annie Goodrich, *The Social and Ethical Significance of Nursing* (New York: Macmillan, 1932); for the earlier discussions in the 1890s, see Janet Wilson James, "Isabel Hampton and the Professionalization of Nursing," in *The Therapeutic Revolution: Essays in the Social History of American Medicine*,

ed. Morris J. Vogel and Charles E. Rosenberg (Philadelphia: University of Pennsylvania Press, 1979), pp. 201–44. The Grading Committee's views are summarized in their final report, *Nursing Schools Today—and Tomorrow.*

16. Grading Committee, *Nurses, Patients, and Pocketbooks,* p. 361; on nursing leaders, see, for example, the biographical sketch of Lucy Ayers, a Rhode Island nursing educator in *Makers of Nursing History,* ed. Meta Pennock (Buffalo: The Lakeside Press, 1949), p. 125. This statement is based on my analysis of ninety identified nationally and locally prominent nursing leaders; see Reverby, "The Nursing Disorder." An attempt to deal with this contradiction can be found in "A Private Duty Dialogue," *AJN* 28 (December 1928): 1217–20.

17. May Ayers Burgess to Elizabeth Burgess, Dec. 29, 1928, Isabel M. Stewart Papers, "Grading Committee" folder, Teachers College Archives, Columbia University, New York, N.Y.

18. "Nurses, Patients and Pocketbooks," read at the Annual Convention of Nursing Organizations, Louisville, Ky., June 7, 1928, and reprinted in *Bulletin of the American Hospital Association* 2 (July 1928): 300.

19. In addition to the requests from nurses, Geister received congratulations for her report from administrators such as E. M. Bluestone and Malcolm MacEachern, physician William Darrach, and nursing philanthropist Frances Payne Bolton. The letters and requests she received in response to her report are in Box 14, Folder 133, Geister Papers. The correspondence and reports by JG cited below are all in the Geister Papers unless otherwise noted; JG to S. Lillian Clayton, July 7, 1928, Box 14, Folder 133; Florence Johnson to JG, Aug. 6, 1926, Box 14, Folder 133; Susan Francis to JG, Oct. 6, 1926, Box 14, Folder 133D.

20. JG, "Biographical Notes," April 1963, Geister inventory file. The biographical material is based on these "Notes." She died in 1964 at the age of seventy-nine.

21. I. S. Falk, "Medical Care in the U.S.A.—1932–1972. Problems, Proposals and Programs from the Committee on the Costs of Medical Care to the Committee for National Health Insurance," *Milbank Memorial Fund Quarterly/Health and Society* 51 (Winter 1973): 3. Falk was describing his fellow members of the Committee on the Costs of Medical Care, but his remarks easily apply to Geister.

22. "Memo to Miss Pennock from Miss Geister," Jan. 20, 1941, Box 10, Folder 89; see also Emilie Sargent to JG, Feb. 15, 1933, Box 15, Folder 139; "Report of October Field Trip—Janet M. Geister, R.N., Nov. 24, 1928," Box 10, Folder 90; see also JG, "Security and Leisure for the Private Duty Nurse," *TNHR* 94 (January 1935): 29–33.

23. JG, "Report of the Committee on the Costs of Medical Care," Memorandum to the Board of Directors, American Nurses' Association, Dec. 2, 1932, Box 10, Folder 90, for the best single explanation of her views on private duty, see "Hearsay and Facts in Private Duty."

24. JG to Mary Thornton Davis, July 15, 1926, Box 14, Folder 133;

Lyda Anderson to JG, May 3, 1930, Box 14, Folder 136; JG to Emilie J. Sargent, Feb. 14, 1931, Box 15, Folder 137.

25. JG, "Abstract of 1933 Program, Part I," submitted to the Board of Directors, American Nurses' Association, December 1932, p. 2, Box 10, Folder 89A. Her political views are clear in JG, "Is the Private Duty Nurse Standing Still?" *TNHR* 98 (January 1937): 31–34, 52; "Abstract of 1933 Program"; "A Challenge to American Nursing," 1934, Box 10, Folder 88; "Visit to Portland to Confer on the Registry Situation," JG Memo to Jane Gavin, March 3, 1930, Box 10, Folder 93; JG to Lyda Anderson, Feb. 2, 1934, Box 15, Folder 140. "Registry Statement," January 26, 1937, Box 10, Folder 89A; "Report of the Committee on the Costs of Medical Care."

26. "Registry Statement"; see also "Abstract of 1933 Program," "A Challenge to American Nursing," "Private Duty Nursing Then–and Now," and JG to Miss [Clara] Quereau, March 9, 1935, Box 15, Folder 141.

On her concern for forging links between private duty nurses and the VNAs, and her awareness of the difficulties, see "Registry Statement," JG to Michael M. Davis, Oct. 14, 1932, Box 15, Folder 138; JG to Emilie G. Sargent, Oct. 16, 1926, Box 14, Folder 133D; JG to Emilie G. Sargent, Feb. 14, 1931, Box 15, Folder 137.

27. "Abstract of 1933 Program," p. 6; Louise Tattershall, "Hourly Nursing in Public Health Nursing Associations," *Public Health Nursing* 19 (August 1927): 397–402; Mary Sewell Gardner, *Public Health Nursing*, 3rd ed. (New York: Macmillan, 1936); M. Louise Fitzpatrick, *The National Organization of Public Health Nursing, 1912–1952, Development of a Practice Field* (New York: National League for Nursing, 1975); Karen Buhler-Wilkerson, "False Dawn: The Rise and Decline of Public Health Nursing in America, 1900–1930" (chap. 5, above).

28. On community nursing, see JG to M. Adelaide Nutting, Aug. 23, 1932, quoted by Theresa Christy, "The First Fifty Years," *AJN* 71 (Sept. 1971): 1781; JG to Michael M. Davis, June 11, 1932, Box 15, Folder 138; "Abstract of 1933 Program," p. 8. Information on the Registry Committee can be found in JG, "History of the Dismissal of the Registry Committee" statement, no date, probably 1934, Box 10, Folder 89A. See also, "Registry Statement"; "Progress Report of the Registry Study," Box 10, Folder 89; "Report of the Registry Committee–1930–1932," Box 10, Folder 92. For reports on registry discussions at the 1930 biennial ANA convention, see *AJN* 30 (July 1930): 827–39. See also, ANA *Board of Directors Minutes*, 1928–34, Boxes 39–41, ANA Papers. Geister quotation on the adjustment of the private duty nurse is in JG, "A Challenge to American Nursing," pp. 8–12.

29. JG to Miss Thomson, Sept. 1, 1932, Box 10, Folder 89A; "Memorandum to the Board of Directors ANA from JG," March 15, 1933 and March 25, 1933, Box 10, Folder 90; JG to Daisy Dean Urch, Feb. 2, 1934, Box 15, Folder 140; Goostray, *Memoirs*, p. 67. The brief report on her "resignation" can be found in the ANA *Board of Directors Minutes*, Jan.

25–30, 1933, p. 41, Box 41, ANA Papers. The board meeting began on Thursday morning, Jan. 25, and Geister's "resignation" came on Monday afternoon, Jan. 30, after many of her supporters on the board had already left. Unfortunately the verbatim minutes of the board for the period 1930–33 were left in "Chicago storage" and never given to the Nursing Archives. This reference is therefore to the published minutes and none of the discussion at the meeting is available.

Geister's view of what she considered to be a "firing" can be found in JG to Emily Hicks, June 6, 1934, Box 15, Folder 140; "Registry Statement"; JG to Lyda Anderson, Oct. 14, 1933; Lyda Anderson to JG, Oct. 16, 1933, Box 15, Folder 139A. See also Ethel Taylor to Major Julia C. Stimson, Feb. 1, 1933, Box 10, Folder 89A. The "understanding Friend" quotation is in Ethel M. Smith to JG, Oct. 16, 1933, Box 15, Folder 139A.

30. My interpretation of the Distribution Committee's work is based on a critical reading of the ANA Board of Directors minutes, the committee reports and minutes, and Geister's criticisms. See, ANA *Board of Directors Minutes*, 1928–35, Boxes 39–42, ANA Papers; "Report of the Committee on the Distribution of Nursing Service, 1930–32," Box 10, Folder 92, Geister Papers; JG, "History of the Dismissal of Registry Committee" statement, Box 10, Folder 89A.

For the official nursing viewpoint, written by the secretary of the committee and the director at headquarters, see Ella Best, *Brief Historical Review and Information About Current Activities of the ANA* (New York: ANA, 1940), 47–55; Emilie Sargent, "The Nursing Profession Works for Recovery," *AJN* 33 (December 1933): 1165–72. Flanagan, *One Strong Voice*, pp. 87–88, has a similar, noncritical viewpoint, which fails to examine the situation below the rhetorical level.

The Director of the Buffalo VNA's quotation is in JG, "Registry Statement"; see also ANA *Board of Directors Minutes*, January 1932, Box 40, ANA Papers. For more on the registry work, see ANA *Board of Directors Minutes*, 1932–35, Boxes 40–42, ANA Papers; JG, "Registry Statement"; "History of the Dismissal of Registry Committee."

31. "Review of Headquarters Activities for 1934 and Suggested Program for 1935," ANA *Board of Directors Minutes*, January 1935, Box 42, ANA Papers; Best, *Brief Historical Review*, pp. 53–54, 58–62; Flanagan, *One Strong Voice*, pp. 105–7. See also the monthly registry reports in the *AJN* and registry surveys in Box 271, ANA Papers.

Roberts, *American Nursing*, pp. 122–24. Roberts places the blame for this situation on nurses' narrow loyalties to their schools and their lack of community-mindedness. Geister is not mentioned. Christy, "The First Fifty Years," p. 1781.

32. Minutes of Meetings of the Community Nursing Service Committee, 1935–40, Box 171, ANA Papers; Best, *Brief Historical Review*, pp. 54–58.

33. Davis, "Nursing Service Measured by Social Needs," p. 36. In an

editorial comment on Davis's challenge ("Needed—More Nursing Service: A Slogan for 1939," *AJN* [January 1939]: 54–55) the editors of the journal seemed to have missed the point of Davis's concern. Their editorial calls for more specialization and better preparation of nurses and applauds the move toward more joint leadership in nursing.

34. JG, "Registry Statement." See also JG, "Is the Private Duty Nurse Standing Still?" p. 35.

35. Gardner, *Public Health Nursing*; NOPHN, *Principles and Practices in Public Health Nursing, Including Cost Analysis* (New York: Macmillan, 1932); NOPHN, *Survey of Public Health Nursing Administration and Practice* (New York: Commonwealth Fund, 1934); Buhler-Wilkerson, "False Dawn."

36. See nn. 26 and 28 above. See also Dorothy Deming, "One Way Out: An Answer to Some Problems of Private Duty Nursing," *Survey*, June 15, 1926, where it is suggested that hourly work should be done by the better-organized VNAs. May Ayers Burgess had the article copied and sent to the members of the Grading Committee, with a note suggesting the problems of public and medical acceptance of visiting nursing and the reluctance of private duty nurses to join the VNAs. May Ayers Burgess to the committee, July 12, 1926, M. Adelaide Nutting Papers, Teachers College Archives, Columbia University, New York, N.Y. The JG quotation is from JG, "Abstract of 1933 Program," p. 4.

37. Davis, "Nursing Service Measured by Social Needs," p. 38.

38. Geister's support letters are in her papers, Box 15, Folders 139 and 140. They came from all over the country and were not just from private duty nurses, as Goostray's comments suggest (see *Memoirs*, p. 67). Her allegations on the political manipulations are in JG to Mrs. August, May 16, 1934, Box 15, Folder 140.

39. She authored over three hundred articles, many of which are in her papers and in the *Trained Nurse*. Her monthly column in the *Trained Nurse* was entitled "Plain Talk." The quotation on laissez-faire policy is from JG to Clara Quereau, March 9, 1935, Box 15, Folder 141. Her views in 1963 are in JG, "Biographical Notes."

40. Jonathan Grossman, *William Sylvis, Pioneer of American Labor* (New York: Columbia University Press, 1945), pp. 191–217; Philip Foner, *Women and the American Labor Movement* (New York: Free Press, 1979), pp. 88, 117–18, 155–56; Daniel Rodgers, *The Work Ethic in America* (Chicago: University of Chicago Press, 1978), pp. 40–45; John R. Commons, et al., *History of Labour in the United States*, 4 vols. (New York: Macmillan, 1921), II, passim; "The Girls' Co-operative Collar Co., *Revolution* 5 (April 28, 1870), p. 267, reprinted in Rosalyn Baxandall, Linda Gordon, and Susan Reverby, eds., *America's Working Women: A Documentary History* (New York: Random House and Vintage, 1976), p. 116. Committee on the Costs of Medical Care, *Medical Care for the American People*, The Final Report of the Committee on the Costs of Medical Care

(Chicago: University of Chicago Press, 1932); Rosemary Stevens, *American Medicine and the Public Interest* (New Haven: Yale University Press, 1971), pp. 175–97.

For examples of the difficulties of reform, see Allon Peebles, et al., *Nursing Services and Insurance for Medical Care in Brattleboro, Vermont* (Chicago: University of Chicago Press, 1932); Falk, Rorem, and Ring, *The Costs of Medical Care*, pp. 476–77; Dorothy F. Johnston, *History and Trends of Practical Nursing* (St. Louis: C. V. Mosby, 1966), pp. 21–24. On the continuing difficulty of patients to pay for private duty services, see Margaret C. Klem, "Who Purchase Private Duty Nursing Services," *AJN* 39 (October 1939): 1069–77. On Waltham, see Alfred Worcester, "The Waltham Nursing Service Bureau," reprint from *Southern Medicine and Surgery* 99 (March 1937), Box 1, Waltham Training School for Nurses Papers, Nursing Archive, Mugar Library, Boston University.

8

Doctors, Patients, and "Big Nurse": Work and Gender in the Postwar Hospital

Barbara Melosh

Women's dominance in nursing nearly equals their monopoly on motherhood: nursing has always been a woman's job. But over the last century that work has undergone dramatic changes in content, setting, and organization. In the mid-nineteenth century, most nursing care was done by women in families. Florence Nightingale's 1860 *Notes on Nursing*, later the sacred text of the nursing profession, was addressed to laywomen; its preface declared, "Every woman is a nurse." As medical care became more complex and more tied to hospitals, nursing gradually separated from the sphere of home and family and became established as paid work that required special training. Still, arguments of women's special fitness continued to link women's participation in this new category of paid work to traditional domestic roles. As one doctor wrote in the 1920s, "A hospital is a home for the sick, and there can be no home . . . unless there is a woman at the head of it." While these sentimental images lingered, the actual practice of nursing grew more specialized. In the esoteric technological setting of modern hospitals, no one would proclaim that "every woman is a nurse." But the cultural ideology of woman's place still informs the medical division of labor: nearly every nurse is a woman.[1]

As a consistently female occupation in a rapidly changing work setting, nursing offers an illuminating example of the ways in which gender informs work, and conversely, how work both reproduces and transforms existing relationships of power and inequality. Medical division of labor replicates a larger sexual division of labor. At work, nurses care for helpless patients and defer to doctors just as women care for children and defer to fathers or husbands in families. But the undeniable structural constraints of nursing have not remained static or uncontested. Rather, nursing has changed under the impact of expanding medical science and technology, with shifts in the organization of health care, and through nurses' own activities and organization. As it developed, this quintessentially "female" job took a historical turn that threatened and disrupted the traditional division of labor.

After 1940 nurses gained a new leverage at work. The growth of medicine expanded their skills, the move from private duty to hospital work enhanced their authority, and the supply of nurses lagged behind the demand of a proliferating health care industry, giving weight to nurses' discontents and demands on the job. As nurses began to claim more control at work and to assume command of an imposing technology, their work increasingly jarred cultural prescriptions for women's place. The disjuncture did not go unremarked. In a postwar society that called for a return to domesticity, nurses' expanded roles were contested and challenged. In the 1940s, 1950s, and 1960s sociological studies, prescriptive literature, and popular fiction all reflected a growing unease with the nurse's expertise and authority. In its revealing portrayals of nurses and of women, this literature documents a cultural history that has been missing from existing interpretations of nursing history.[2]

Nurses' experience is a compelling case study of the complex relationships of gender and work in the twentieth century, one that suggests new insights for women's history, labor history, and medical history. And yet nursing history has seldom been viewed from the vantage point of any of these perspectives. A rich body of literature, written by nurses themselves, has recounted the internal development of the occupation. Cast in the framework and ideology of professionalization, these narratives dramatize a history of progress, from "the twilight and the darkness" before Nightingale to the triumphs of reform, reorganization, and upgraded education. This perspective has provided a useful outline for the institutional history of nursing, which these authors helped to shape in their own careers, and it reveals much about the accomplishments, motivations, and aspirations of women like them, nursing's elite. But the very visibility of these vocal and articulate leaders has obscured the experience and consciousness of other nurses. Leaders' rhetoric of professionalization has set the boundaries of discussion and analysis of nurses and nursing: even those historians and sociologists who argue that nursing is *not* a profession still view professional ideology or "professionalism" as the shaping force in nurses' consciousness as workers. Similarly most women's historians and labor historians have overlooked nursing altogether, consigning it to the purview of the professions and thus beyond the scope of their own search for the data of ordinary people's work and lives.[3]

Historians of nursing must move beyond the limiting framework of professionalization to locate nurses as women and as workers. In doing so we move from an internal portrayal of nursing toward a revision informed by the broader concerns of social history: an interpretation set in the context of women's changing prospects and life choices, attentive to the history of medicine and to the special character of medical workplaces, infused with the labor historian's sense of the structure and experience of work.

In turn, as historians engaged in this task we have much to bring to the fields that are nourishing our reformulation of nursing history. Too often I sense in our own discussions and presentations a note of apology that suggests too narrow a view of what we are about. We fall into the tacit assumption that nursing history will remain a separate field, improved by the insights of social history but not a vital part of it. I think we should abandon this deference for a more active sense of the dialectical relationship between subject and method. Nurses are workers in an occupation that has consistently employed large numbers of women; in the medical division of labor, nursing occupies a key position that has been largely overlooked in medical history and sociology; it provides a significant example of a major service industry over a century when such work has come to dominate the economy and the labor force. As we bring the questions of medical history, women's history, and labor history to the data of nurses' experience, we shall revise and challenge these formulations even as we forge a stronger and more comprehensive nursing history.

After 1940 changes both inside and outside the workplace set the conflicts between traditional female domesticity and women's paid work into sharp relief. Nurses began to enjoy a favorable labor market for the first time in decades as administrators began to fill their expanding wards with graduates, revising hospitals' long-standing dependence on the labor of apprentice student nurses. In 1927 nearly three-quarters of hospitals with training schools had relied exclusively on students for ward nursing services; a decade later most reported that they had begun to employ some graduate staff nurses. By 1940 nearly half of all nurses were employed in hospitals, and by the end of World War II hospital jobs claimed a decisive majority of active nurses. The nurses' employment crisis of the 1920s eased as hospitals hired more graduates through the

1930s, and evaporated altogether with mobilization for war. Hospitals needed nurses' skills and labor, and after the war they urgently recruited women to remedy the shortage that has persisted into the present.[4]

The content and organization of hospital work bolstered nurses' efforts to define and defend their skills. First, expanding opportunities in hospitals relocated nurses in institutional workplaces, which improved their positions relative to doctors and revised their old dependence on the patient as employer. Second, both the shortage of nurses and the expansion of medical therapeutics lent a new legitimacy to nursing. A climate of scarcity and the performance of complicated tasks combined to support nurses' long-standing claims to special expertise. In the 1920s nurses had suffered the insecurity of the declining market of private duty, and grown increasingly restive with the galling personal service associated with that work. By the 1940s they triumphantly assumed positions of middle management and recognized technical skill in hospitals.

At the head of the medical division of labor, doctors had always set the limits of nurses' authority and held the right to control the content of their work. Nurses' transition to the hospital did not overturn the ironclad rule of medical dominance: by law and custom doctors were nurses' superiors. Nonetheless, these relationships changed as nurses moved from private duty into hospital work. The conditions of an institutional workplace imposed new constraints on physicians' exercise of authority and simultaneously created a favorable setting for nurses to expand their own sphere.

The economic and social arrangements of hospital work lessened the physician's direct control over nurses' employment. In free-lance work nurses needed doctors' referrals to get and keep cases. A doctor who disliked a private duty nurse's methods, her manner, or even her appearance could get her fired quickly. The nurse had no protection against such arbitrary practices, and no recourse. Hospital nurses might still risk their jobs by repeatedly irritating or challenging a powerful doctor, but because they were hired by the institution, they were no longer directly dependent on the goodwill of any one physician.

The bureaucratic structure of the hospital diffused medical authority, and offered nurses a modicum of support when conflicts arose with physicians. Medical practice operated under new constraints in the hospital. Doctors worked under the eyes of their peers and were subject, at least nominally, to the supervision and discipline of the medical chief of staff. The more public character of hospital work limited the physician's absolute authority. The private duty nurse who questioned a doctor faced the consequences alone. In the hospital a doubtful nurse could appeal to other knowledgeable participants, or invoke the impersonal authority of bureaucratic procedures and policies. Conflicts between nurses and doctors were still weighted in favor of physicians, yet nurses gained a new leverage. Hospital nurses had the support of small work groups, and the resource of a formal structure of appeal. Buttressed by her head nurse and sympathetic colleagues, a nurse could more readily confront a doctor on the floor. If informal approaches failed she could take the conflict through established channels and seek arbitration through the higher authorities of the nursing director and the chief physician. Such bureaucracies did not automatically guarantee even-handed treatment, but they did provide nurses with a hearing. The acute shortage of nurses and their important place in the hospital also meant that administrators had a new stake in defending them. In one example several surgical nurses resigned in protest against the hospital's irascible surgeons. The administrator persuaded them to stay and called in the medical chief of staff to discipline the doctors. " 'We just can't afford to lose good nurses like that. You're going to have to tell them to lay off.' " Such incidents probably remained exceptional, yet that they occurred at all testified to the benefits of nurses' new market positions.[5]

Hospital nurses occupied strategic positions in the institution. The nurse commanded the domain of her ward: she knew how to negotiate the red tape of hospital rules, placate the patients, and get the work done. Learning to win the nurse's loyalty was part of an intern's initiation, and medical lore wryly acknowledged nurses' pivotal roles. A good nurse, every physician knew, could smooth his way as well as make his work more effective. Formally, of course, the nurse's duty was still to obey the doctor. But doctors who tried to enforce their prerogatives too insistently might find themselves stymied at every turn. Very secure nurses might risk the aggressive strategy of "forgetting" or simply ignoring a problematic order. In a safer and probably more common tactic, nurses could effectively hamstring a difficult doctor by working to rule: bringing him to the hospital at all hours by refusing verbal orders, invoking esoteric rules and procedures, inciting rebellion among his patients by refusing to discuss his plans or methods. Some obdurate doctors might persist in their folly, but most found it simpler to bend somewhat to the nurse's authority over the ward.[6]

Moreover the new content of medical care made nursing and medical work more interdependent. As advances in surgical and medical techniques promoted more aggressive medical intervention, the nurse's close observation became critical in the treatment of very sick patients. The polio epidemic of the late 1940s offered a dramatic example, as illustrated in one nurse's account. With careful observation, she detected a minute change in a young woman's breathing. Recognizing this as a sign of impending paralysis, she quickly called the attending doctor. The patient was placed in an iron lung, where she eventually recovered. Nurses had always been responsible for close observation of their patients, and good nursing care had often determined the outcome in diseases like typhoid fever, scarlet fever, diphtheria, and pneumonia in the days before antibiotic therapy. But the development of new medical technology gave a new significance to nursing care and observation that brought nursing and medicine into a closer alliance on the job. Twenty-five years before, when iron lungs were not yet in use, the nurse's observation would have signaled the limits of medical care; the physician could only watch helplessly and wait to pronounce the patient's death. Such moments had a very different meaning and character as the possibilities for medical intervention expanded. Doctors depended on skilled nurses to watch for critical changes in their absence, and sometimes to initiate emergency treatment themselves. In this situation of close collaboration, doctors had to treat nurses more like medical colleagues.[7]

Nowhere was this more apparent than in the mushrooming special care units. As sophisticated technology supported more elaborate interventions, hospitals began to organize separate units to make more effective use of specialized equipment and personnel. Postoperative care, once provided by special duty nurses or staff nurses on wards throughout the hospital, began to move to recovery rooms where patients were treated until they revived from anesthesia. Medical and surgical intensive care units segregated the sickest patients for concentrated care. By 1960 the term "progressive patient care" indicated the spreading use of this organization: patients migrated through intensive care, intermediate "step-down" units, and regular floor care; or moved from surgery to recovery room to their floors. These changes produced new nursing specialties as nurses followed the proliferation of medical specialties and began to label themselves as intensive care, nephrology, or coronary care nurses. In these settings, nurses assumed many functions and responsibilities formerly reserved for physicians, and claimed a new authority by virtue of their expertise. The pace and character of intensive care left no room for the old formulas of nursing deference. No critical care nurse would call a doctor to report meekly, "Mr. James's pulse appears to have ceased." She would yell for emergency equipment, pound and compress the patient's chest, inflate his lungs, perhaps even begin to administer powerful drugs used in resuscitation. In their turn doctors recognized and relied on the skills and judgment of these nurses.[8]

Hospital employment also dramatically increased nurses' authority with patients. In managing the tasks and relationships of patient care, nurses had long recognized the advantages of the hospital as a workplace. Although free-lancers shunned hospital staff jobs, they preferred to nurse their private cases in the hospital. In the 1920s and 1930s registries complained that they could not find nurses for home patients; private nurses would refuse these cases to hold out for hospital special duty. While the nurse at home had to find a precarious niche for herself in the routines and relationships of the household, the hospital special worked in an environment tailored to medical and nursing routines. This setting tacitly reinforced nurses' legitimacy as skilled workers. They could more closely restrict their duties to specific nursing skills: hospitalized patients could not assign their nurses to cooking, mending, laundry, or child care, as home patients often did. Away from home, patients lost other familiar resources and prerogatives, and nurses gained an unprecedented social control. Hospitalized patients depended on their nurses to negotiate a threatening and unfamiliar world—to bring them meals and linen, to deliver messages, to admit visitors. The impressive technological apparatus of nursing and medicine underscored the nurse's claim to special expertise. In vivid contrast to their uneasy charges, nurses were insiders, initiates into the mysterious workings of the hospital. Private duty patients still retained the last prerogative of employers, and they could fire an unsatisfactory nurse. But short of this final authority, patients had lost much of their former power to define the content and practice of nurses' work.[9]

General duty nurses slipped altogether beyond the reaches of the private duty patient's dwindling authority, for they were employed by the hospital, not by the patient. Institutional nursing released nurses from the vestiges of personal service that clung to private duty. As one grateful ex-private duty nurse commented, " 'I don't have to entertain the patient and help trim last year's hat!' " Responsible for more than one patient, the nurse could limit the demands of any one person and, working together, nurses developed and enforced a shared prescription for the "good" patient. By disciplining patients to their proper roles, nurses avoided many of the disadvantages of private duty and could negotiate some respite from the quickening pace of hospital work. The well-schooled patient did not waste nursing time with trivialities.[10]

Finally nurses secured their positions at the head of a nursing hierarchy that became more clearly and rigidly defined in the postwar years. As hospitals grew in the late 1930s and 1940s and as costs increased steadily, nursing leaders gradually yielded to hospital administrators' and public pressure for formal definition and training of a subsidiary nurse, a worker who could do some of the registered nurse's tasks for less money. The war years accelerated this growing division of labor. Military nursing provided a dramatic model for a fully rationalized work force, and placed the graduate nurse at the head of it. Commissioned as second lieutenants, nurses had regular rank for the first time. In the services they enjoyed the privileges of officers, and on the ward they were the supervisors and military superiors of medical corpsmen and the enlisted men who were their patients. At home the widespread use of Red Cross volunteer aides and paid subsidiary workers forced nurses to define their own skills and to develop ways to use and supervise auxiliaries. After the war nursing leaders moved to ratify and control the emerging division of labor, joining the hospitals and the young National Association for Practical Nurses' Education to formulate accrediting standards. During the 1950s licensing laws passed in state after state.[11]

Rationalization created a middle-management role for nurses. As charge nurses responsible for a shift or as head nurses who ran a whole floor, they moved from the bedside to supervisory and administrative positions. They kept records, managed workers under them, coordinated treatment plans, made out shift schedules, followed up orders. Responsible to both administrators and physicians, nurses occupied a critical position in the hospital. As middle managers, they mediated between bureaucratic demands for order and efficiency and the more chaotic universe of patients' needs and physicians' individual styles of treatment.

If nurses confronted a wider range of possibilities in the hospital, they were still far from claiming real control over their work. General duty nurses were bitterly aware of the constraints of their new relationship to administrators. Some former private duty nurses experienced hospital employment as a loss of personal independence and cherished craft control. Many disliked the new division of labor, protesting the definition of bedside nursing as less skilled work. On the job nurses resisted speed-up and challenged management's definitions of efficient work. Charge nurses and head nurses chafed under new mountains of paperwork and complained of the frustrations of heavy medical and administrative demands, overcrowded wards, and understaffing. Facing the pressure and pace of hospital work, nurses may well have wondered if they had stopped being the servants of private duty patients only to become the slaves of administrators.[12]

Whatever the real limitations on hospital nurses' work, though, they had gained enough expertise and authority to threaten cultural prescriptions for women. Nurses' increasing skill and influence placed them on a collision course with the postwar ideology of domesticity later named "the feminine mystique." Sources as diverse as nursing manuals, sociological studies, and popular fiction all revealed a heightened concern with nurses as women, a new sense of the possible contradictions and conflicts between the demands of work and the claims of gender. After 1940 portrayals of nursing in prescriptive literature and fiction often showed nurses as failed women, sometimes pathetic, sometimes dangerous in their distance from proper female activities and aspirations. In this pervasive theme postwar observers registered the changes in nurses' work and warned of its pernicious effects on female character.

The outpouring of advice, analyses, and fiction about nurses creates a revealing and variegated resource for the social and cultural historian. Written for different purposes and audiences, these sources must be read with sensitivity to their particular forms and meanings. But each provides an angle of vision that helps to sharpen and widen our views of nursing in the postwar years.

Some wrote directly to an audience of nurses, prospective nurses, or lay persons concerned about nursing. Ethics or professional-adjustments manuals, sociological studies of nursing, and didactic fiction about nurses all focused specifically on nurses' positions in the postwar world, both at work and at home. Such sources provide insight into the contemporary discussion of nursing needs, perceptions, and judgments about changes in nurses' work, and the initiatives and responses of nursing leaders in this situation. All of this literature was intended as prescriptive literature. Nursing manuals and didactic novels were written by nurses or by allies who shared their goals. The manuals directly discuss proper professional and ethical conduct, and all give some attention to the nurse as a woman. Although sociological studies are not conventionally described as prescriptive, the term seems appropriate for postwar studies about nursing. Many were sponsored by policymaking groups or foundations, and many were motivated specifically by the concern for the postwar nursing shortage. Many end in specific recommendations for the reorganization of nursing, and all contain implicit models of good nurses and effective nursing.

Didactic novels represent a special form of prescriptive literature. I classify a novel about nurses as didactic fiction when the author's primary intention appears to be to present an exemplary nurse, to purvey a favorable image of nursing, or to recruit young women into the profession. Most of them are directed to teenage girls, an audience that nurses and concerned lay persons were eager to reach. Nurses themselves wrote many of these novels, turning to the vehicle of fiction in an effort to broaden the audience for their message. This category overlaps with the larger and more general category of fiction using nurse characters. But I have assigned it a separate label to emphasize the special intentions and self-consciousness of these authors.

The authors of most fiction plied their craft with a different intention and another audience in mind. Few, if any, were bent on making a statement about nurses and nursing as such. And yet nurses were perennially popular characters in the pages of their short stories and novels. The gripping drama of the hospital setting makes it an enduring subject of fiction. At times nurses simply serve to fill out the cast of stories and novels with a medical theme; at other times they take center stage. Indeed by the 1950s nurses began to claim a whole genre of their own. Avid readers and booksellers recognized it as such: one can walk into many a used bookstore or public library to find a section devoted to "nurse-romances."

Taken together, didactic novels about nurses, fiction with nurse characters, and genre literature about nursing comprise a large literature. This analysis of fictional portrayals of nurses and nursing is based on my readings of over one hundred novels and short stories containing nurse characters. I compiled titles of novels from several editions of the *Fiction Index* and used similar bibliographical aids to find short stories. Pulp fiction and genre literature can be elusive if one confines the search to traditional scholarly sources, for these titles are not included in the standard reference works and not systematically collected by most libraries. On the other hand, they are abundantly available in the haunts of their followers (and I certainly count myself among the faithful): garage sales, Salvation Army stores, and mass-market outlets like grocery-store fiction racks. Because much fiction about nurses comes from sources beyond the reach of systematic cataloguing, counting, or collecting, nothing resembling a systematic sample can be identified. Since there is no reliable way to delimit the sample, I have not attempted any quantitative content analysis but, rather, have relied on traditional literary methods of close reading and interpretation.

Recognizing the special character of fiction, historians often hesitate to use it as a source. Of course we cannot read fiction as a direct transcription of prevailing cultural ideology: authors filter and necessarily reorder the reality they perceive. But the very act of transformation is what gives fiction its value as a source of cultural history. In analyzing fiction, I look to see how nurse characters are represented, where they stand in the moral universe of the fiction, why the authors select nurses to carry forward the narrative, the metaphors, the message of the fiction.

For genre literature the task is less complex. A few stock plots leap out at the most unwitting reader, and the historian's work is then to analyze the structure and the variations as one piece of the cultural ideology that shapes and informs our lives, whether or not we are readers of fiction. I do not assume that any one short story or novel, however popular, represents *the* public image of nursing but, rather, I look within the fiction for the underlying assumptions, the common culture it draws on, that base of language and ideology that writers must touch to engage their readers. As cultural texts, short stories and novels can tell us much about women's work and women's place in the twentieth century.

American culture has never given more than a reluctant and partial assent to the notion of women in the paid labor force, though more and more women entered it over the twentieth century. During World War II the needs of a defense economy strained but did not shatter time-honored conceptions of women's proper place. Although vigorous recruitment campaigns proclaimed women's fitness for work previously reserved for men, wartime propaganda never failed to note that women were called just "for the duration." Like other women, nurses were recruited in the name of their traditional relationships to men. Over and over wartime rhetoric reminded the nurse that she was on the job as "the ambassador of all we left behind . . . our own mother, wife, sweetheart, or daughter." And even as nurses took on military rank with the responsibilities of command and the hardships of both domestic and foreign service, observers who commended their courage also insistently portrayed their femininity. As a sentimental male historian of nursing wrote in 1946, "Femininity in foxholes, with mud-caked khaki coveralls over pink panties, captured the imagination of the public and fighting men of America." Once an Allied victory seemed assured, plans to restore the normal order shifted into gear. As the defense industry converted to consumer production, women in those highly visible jobs lost them to returning veterans.[13]

But like most of the women who worked in World War II, nurses did not go home. Throughout the 1950s, even as the back-to-the-home movement dominated popular culture and prescriptive literature, more and more women surged into the expanding service sector. Increasingly, too, women combined family responsibilities and paid work, as attested by the rising number of married women and mothers on the job. Located in the burgeoning hospital industry, nurses experienced the contradictions of the feminine mystique in an especially acute and visible form. Hospitals pleaded for them to stay as the nursing shortage grew to crisis dimensions. National recruitment campaigns urged young women into nursing schools and pressed inactive nurses to return to work. At the same time other sources warned nurses that work and womanhood posed conflicting and irreconcilable demands.[14]

The most negative depictions of nursing suggested that the authority of the nurse's position was anomalous and unnatural, distorting female personality into a new and threatening posture of dominance. A curious sociological study, Richard R. Lanese's *Authoritarianism in Nurses*, illustrates the troubled attention to women as nurses. "Authoritarianism" was a word much bandied about in the 1940s and 1950s as a spate of literature took up and popularized the Frankfurt School's concern with the sources of fascism. Deeply shaken by the rise of fascism in Europe and repelled by Stalinism in the Soviet Union, Americans identified both the right and the left with totalitarianism. In one manifestation of this pervasive concern, Lanese argued that the hospital environment attracted and fostered "authoritarian personalities." He purported to measure nurses' authoritarian leanings with the since discredited "F-scale," designed to diagnose and prevent tendencies toward fascism. Although his data failed to support his major hypothesis, he concluded somewhat limply, "[N]evertheless, the variable [authoritarianism] appears to be a significant attitude and personality dimension among the nurses sampled." The selection of nurses as a focus for this study strikingly illustrates the postwar attack on working women. More powerful doctors or administrators were surely more prone to abuse of authority than nurses. But as women in some semblance of command, nurses were both more visible and more threatening.[15]

In fiction sentimental images of angels in white yielded to more unsettling if also more colorful characters. "Hot Lips," the crack surgical nurse in M*A*S*H, ran her nurses with an iron hand and kept the irreverent doctors and enlisted men at a respectful distance. The formidable "Big Nurse" of Ken Kesey's *One Flew Over the Cuckoo's Nest* (1962) policed her male patients to enforce her own version of order and discipline on the mental ward. In characterizations like these the hospital world reordered the accustomed hierarchy of gender. Nurse characters gained a new and disquieting power as their skills and authority at work reversed the proper dominance of men over women.

Novels and short stories often showed male patients at the mercy of their nurses, using the cultural anomaly of female authority to shape literary metaphors. In an especially striking example, a short story published in 1956 portrays a patient's relationship with his nurse to represent the frightening dependence and isolation of physical disability. T. K.

Brown's prize-winning "A Drink of Water" explores the plight of a soldier who has lost his sight, his arms, and his legs in an explosion. While the fastidious critic or squeamish reader might rebel at this excess, the extreme situation of Fred MacCann effectively underscores the patient's vulnerability. Fred must depend on his nurses to supply all his physical needs, to inform him about his surroundings, and indeed to mediate most of his action in the world. A gentle nurse gradually brings Fred out of his despair and grief. While not too bright, she is good at anticipating his needs—to all appearances, in short, your ideal woman. Inevitably Fred comes to adore the hands and voice that have saved him.

The plot gains momentum as the nurse unexpectedly reciprocates and approaches him sexually. Delirious with surprise and gratitude, Fred finds himself in a torrid affair, and the two occupy their days in circumventing narrow-minded hospital authorities to drink and carry on in Fred's room. But one night the motherly-nurse-turned-seducer reveals yet another side of herself. To his horror she breathes heavily into his ear and calls him her "man-thing." He realizes bitterly that the nurse's desire is not the affirmation of his intact humanity but, rather, the ultimate objectification: to her he is only "a phallus on its small pedestal of flesh." He probes her past to confirm his dark suspicions. Just as he had feared, his beloved is a "man-hater": she can only love a helpless and mutilated man. Devastated, he kills himself, an act requiring no little ingenuity under the circumstances. In a world turned upside down, men lose their power to women, and women with unnatural power abuse it.[16]

This thread runs through postwar popular culture about nurses. Nurse characters unbalance the proper relationships between men and women, alternately ordering men about and ignoring them; often asserting an unseemly sexual autonomy either by seducing male patients or by abandoning them altogether for celibacy or lesbianism. The titillating novel *Night Nurse*, published by Venus Books, provides a convenient example in its transparent exploitation of this theme. In the plot, work becomes the vehicle for nurse Kathy's sexual revenge on men. Seduced and abandoned by a rich hometown boy, Kathy claims independence by throwing herself into work and withholding her sexuality.

> Nursing became her passion, and gradually she got the reputation of being a cold woman, an inhuman thing who had ice in her veins.
>
> She became proud of this, and tried all the harder to subjugate her emotions. She would be impervious to men, unfettered by the weakness of sex. It would be her strength. Through it she would have the power to hurt men as Ken had hurt her.

In order to implement this vengeance most efficiently, she volunteers for an all-male ward. Beautiful but untouchable (or as the author would have it, "temptation dressed in white"), Kathy gloats at the prospect of provoking and then rejecting the advances of her helpless male patients. "She would be able to taunt them, to laugh at them, to treat them impersonally like dogs." The plot predictably follows Kathy's conversion from this unwomanly position. After a provocative resistance, she succumbs to the advances of one of her patients. Male sexuality triumphantly overcomes the nurse's defiant distance, a moment immortalized with a torrent of soft-porn clichés. "As though she were compelled by a force outside herself, her lips came down against his. . . ." "She was like clay in his hands. . . ." "He was a tempting, desirable lamp that she fluttered around, mothlike, unable to escape!"[17]

In part such tales simply elaborate on the time-worn identification of nurses with forbidden sexuality. In its persistence and power this theme touches deeper cultural sources than postwar social and economic changes alone. Nurses' historical precedents still faintly color perceptions of the work. In the nineteenth century nursing was often associated with prostitution as female nurses followed the army with their less reputable sisters. In peacetime nurses also suffered guilt by association with female hospital attendants who came from prisons. More immediately the physical intimacy of nursing evokes sexual associations that feed into the stock character of lustful or too-knowing nurses. The portrayal of nurses' sexuality might also be interpreted in the larger cultural dichotomy posed in images of the Virgin and the whore; like other women, nurses appear either as saintly angels or as degraded creatures of the flesh.

Postwar fiction on nursing undoubtedly taps these longer roots, but the characterizations do bring a new twist to the nurse's legendary sexual expertise. In earlier depictions nursing is shown as marginal work done by marginal women: on the edges of social life, sexual license becomes broader and deviance finds its own niche. Postwar fiction alters the formula by showing competent nurses as questionable women. Once shown as the embodiment of idealized female character, nursing increasingly appears as work that would pervert or unsex women. An excerpt from one sociological interview offers telling evidence for this interpretation. In response to the question "How are nurses different from other women?" the male informant replied, " 'I'd rather not say. Oh, some nurses are okay, but you know yourself what they are like.' [Interviewer: 'No, what?'] 'Well, a young nurse has spent a lot of time on her education and she feels like she is somebody and you can't tell me they don't get out and find out what things are all about.' " In depictions like this, nursing is threatening not because it is marginal work, but because it gives women too much control.[18]

Popular fiction, didactic novels, and prescriptive literature all reflected a new sense of the conflicting demands of work and womanhood. The fiction warned that commitment to work imperiled women's social and emotional lives. The common stereotype of the head nurse or supervisor showed nurses with authority as frustrated single women, battle-axes who might be respected but were not loved. In one unsubtle version, a co-worker presses home the message. " 'Tremendous nurse,' " he comments. " 'She has nothing to distract her from her work. I just wonder . . . what does she do after she leaves this place? After she's fed the cat and cleaned the canary's cage?' " The young nurses in another novel shudder at the life of their dedicated supervisor. " 'She hasn't got a friend outside [the hospital], and half the time she stops on duty because she can't think of anything else to do.' " Competence, altruism, and devotion to duty are all potentially suspect, evidences of incomplete women. Even when such characters are portrayed more sympathetically, they do not provide appealing models. In a sentimental *Saturday Evening Post* story, the strict nurse dubbed "Old Ironpuss" turns out to have a heart of gold. Her sternness provides a necessary edge: deliberately she provokes patients' anger to distract them from self-pity and to stir their efforts to recover. She sacrifices love and companionship to establish needed discipline for her patients and staff. While the portrait is admiring, it hardly inspires emulation. "Old Ironpuss" is a good nurse because she is an eccentric: she can accept the harsh discipline of social isolation and asexuality.[19]

In a study of the nurse's personality, the wisdom of social science echoed the literary depiction of nurses as failed women. Condescending and subtly critical, Hans O. Mauksch characterized his composite nursing student as immature, that damning epithet of the 1950s and 1960s: "She would like to be close to people but prefers to avoid final and ultimate responsibility. She seeks the warmth and gratification of the maternal role without fully having to raise the child; she longs for contact with the opposite sex while fearing the consequences of her sexuality." In this analysis of nurses' psychology, the author implied that work provided a kind of surrogate womanhood, a retreat for those unable to meet the challenges of being Real Women.[20]

Genre literature and didactic fiction both revealed the heightened pressure on working women. A common stock plot explored the dilemma of a young nurse poised between professional commitment and postwar womanhood. A heightened concern with "femininity" pervaded novels with nurse protagonists. In one nurse-romance written in 1964 young Taffy chafes at the demands of nursing and envies the regular hours, lighter demands, and more glamorous work settings of her roommates, a secretary and an aspiring actress. Her "sexless" work role disrupts her social life. In one of many such low moments she consults the wisdom of popular songs, remembering the "ribbons and laces and smell of cologne" of "The Girl That I Marry." Against this standard, Taffy admits defeat: "Never a girl in a stiff white uniform, smelling of antiseptic and toting bedpans and sterilizing instruments." A 1949 novel, *Wilderness Nurse*, portrays the problems of a dissatisfied nurse with more realism and complexity, but when Denise decides to leave nursing, she too rejects the nurse's austerity for more "feminine" work: "I want to wear pretty clothes all the time, instead of the eternal white uniform. . . . I want to sit down at a desk. If I stand up to work, say behind a counter, I want to handle nylon stockings or pure-dye silk blouses instead of soiled linen and heavy trays." In these stories nursing undermines female personality, and many a protagonist has moments when she longs to be "a girl instead of a starched robot."[21]

Although nursing often earns the epithet of "unfeminine," it still retains a hold on many fictional protagonists. In these plots, the narrative interest often centers on the fateful lure of work. As surgical nurse Jane Arden muses in a typical reverie, ". . . perhaps she put too much of herself into her work. Perhaps there was not enough left over for a real life, aside from her chosen career, a home of her own, her own man, her own children. Every girl wanted these things more than anything else. Jane was sure that she was no different from other girls; it was just that she was in no hurry to give up nursing." Male suitors or advisers must set these women straight. Nurses who become deeply involved in work soon run into serious conflicts with their boyfriends. In *Tired Feet*, a memoir written as a novel, the nurse refused to leave her work to move to the city where her fiancé lives. He breaks off the engagement and leaves her with these parting words: " '. . . when and if you decide whether it's me you want or your beloved profession, you know where I will be. Goodby!' " When a nurse in another novel breaks a date to assist in emergency surgery, her boyfriend explodes, " 'Serves me right for falling for a girl who isn't a real girl—just a trained nurse robot hypnotized by the doctor.' " In these stock plots nurses come to a hard moment of truth as they recognize that serious work disrupts romance. Most end by accepting the wisdom offered in one novel's pointed scene. A rash young nurse exclaims, " '. . . nursing is the most rewarding profession any woman could hope to know.' " Her mentor, a fatherly physician, amends reprovingly, " 'The second most rewarding. Marriage and motherhood come first.' " The novels typically end with connubial bliss on the horizon, and maintain a discreet silence about whether or not the nurse will continue to work.[22]

All of these stories operate on the implicit assumption that the claims of work and love are mutually exclusive, following the conventions of the feminine mystique and at the same time, of course, obscuring the realities of more and more working women's lives. In their most prominent messages, then, these novels serve to reinforce the verities of the feminine mystique. But the fiction also betrays an ambivalence that often subtly modifies or undercuts their docile resolutions.

Although the stories typically end by endorsing the choice of love, the fictional nurses do not relinquish all their claims to work. The plots set up their protagonists to choose between love and work; but as a reward for their emotional struggle they often win both. In the happy devices of popular fiction, many protagonists manage to reconcile these seemingly conflicting choices. Boyfriends who sulk and threaten when nurses must work cause much heartbreak, but significantly they do not get their women. In *Wilderness Nurse*, Denise at first capitulates and leaves her job, but in the end she returns and defends her work heatedly: ". . . quit running down my profession, the work I like to do best in the world, the work I'll never give up. You'll have to take me on my own terms as a nurse and a—a companion, or not at all. I'm going back to Holland Hospital tomorrow morning."[23]

Frequently nurses discard a petulant layman, often a frivolous rich boy, to find true love with a struggling young doctor who understands the demands of hospital life and shares the nurse's commitment to it. In another solution Sue Barton fends off her suitor for several volumes of the series, successfully withstanding the threat of losing her man to explore more possibilities in her nursing. She marries her loyal doctor when *she* is ready. The eternally single Cherry Ames adroitly evades any serious entanglements, while enjoying the admiration of a string of love-struck men on each assignment. In the harsher scenes of everyday life such easy solutions undoubtedly eluded many women. But the novels ultimately did affirm work in ways that may have moderated the familiar pressure for domesticity.

Prescriptive literature also strained to accommodate professional commitment to the insistent demands of the feminine mystique. One 1947 manual addressed a new question: "Must nurses lose their femininity?" Its description of nurses' goals showed a sharp erosion of this literature's traditional affirmation of the rewards of disciplined work.

"We want to be efficient in our work," the authors asserted feebly, and went on to advise young nurses to strive to be "natural (in the sense of not being strained or affected) . . . pleasing in appearance and manner, and sufficiently feminine to inspire true love in a worthy man." A feature article in *Nursing World* set out a new kind of model with "A Day in the Life of Miss June Reynolds, Senior Nursing Student and 1950 Campus Queen." In the same journal a 1959 column directed readers to seek the delicate balance of "the feminine principle of feeling" versus "the thinking characteristics associated with the masculine principle." The author noted that nurses' education and rising skills were moving nurses closer to the "masculine principle," and warned that "When the feminine side is overwhelmed and pushed into the background, the prevailing symptoms are depression, general dissatisfaction, and lack of zest." The column did not advocate a retreat from the "masculine" aspects of work, but it did present their pitfalls rather vividly. At best the womanly nurse faced a precarious juggling act in managing "male" work and "female" personality.[24]

Both fiction and prescriptive literature struggled to resolve the perceived conflict between work and femininity by reverting to old arguments of women's special fitness for nursing. Lucile Petry, a nursing educator, suggested: "Since it is woman's part to create and heal and comfort, nursing is one of the most rewarding vocations open to women." In this vision work even improved on nature. Petry continued: "Preparation for nursing is more than preparation for a professional career; it is preparation for living as an intelligent citizen, as wife and homemaker." This view of women's education accommodated both the demands of the feminine mystique and the postwar enthusiasm for "life-adjustment" education. It appeared everywhere. One novelist used the depiction of a nursing school commencement to get the message across. The speaker declares, " 'When we educate a man . . . we educate an individual; but when we educate a woman, we educate a family.' " In the audience, an approving man assents, " 'Perfect preparation for wife and motherhood.' " When one of Cherry Ames's suitors begs for her hand, he says coyly, " 'I've heard tell that nurses make the best wives and mothers.' " Nurses trained in the 1940s and 1950s remembered hearing this justification again and again. At a time when nurses' work had become far removed from its domestic origins, when nurses on the job were exercising new skills and authority, and when hospitals and patients desperately needed nurses, these revived arguments of special fitness served to defend nursing as proper women's work.[25]

After 1940 nurses' skills and authority increasingly exceeded the limits of acceptable women's work. The threat of this expansion was reflected in postwar imagery that depicted nurses as women who over-stepped the boundaries of appropriate female behavior. Without the defense of an articulate feminist ideology or the support of an active women's movement, nurses often met this attack with rhetorical efforts to accommodate their work to the demands of the feminine mystique. At the same time, though, their experiences and activities in hospitals signaled a developing challenge to the limits of "women's" work. In in-formal negotiations on the job hospital nurses improved their positions with doctors and patients. In a spurt of organization in the late 1940s some general duty nurses took their grievances with administrators to unions, and their militance pushed the reluctant American Nurses' Asso-ciation to represent nurses in collective bargaining. Ultimately, acting in the context of a revived women's movement, nurses would link their grievances as workers to a new consciousness and criticism of their posi-tions as women. But well before the resurgence of feminism, changes in work itself had unsettled the precarious logic of the sexual division of labor; and as nurses pressed the advantages of their new workplace, they had already begun to strain against the deeply entrenched structure of sex segregation itself.

NOTES

This article is a revised and expanded version of material that appears in the introduction and chapter 5 of Melosh, *"The Physician's Hand": Work Culture and Conflict in American Nursing* (Philadelphia: Temple University Press, 1982). I acknowledge gratefully the helpful comments presented at the Rockefeller Conference on Nursing History, May 1981, by Charles Rosenberg and Janet Wilson James. For close reading and useful criticism, I also want to thank Susan Porter Benson, Patricia Cooper, Audrey Davis, Ellen Condliffe Lagemann, Thomas McCormick, Judith Smith, and Deborah Warner. The research was supported by the American Associa-tion of University Women and the Smithsonian Institution.

1. Alfred Worcester, *Nurses and Nursing* (Cambridge: Harvard Uni-versity Press, 1927), p. 9.

2. In "The Proletarianization of Nursing in the United States, 1932–1946," David Wagner argues the opposite case, contending that nurses lost skill in the move from private duty to hospitals. See *International Journal of Health Services* 10 (1980): 271–90. For other discussions of the impact of hospital-based work, see Susan Reverby, "The Search for the Hospital Yard-stick: Nursing and the Rationalization of Hospital Work," in *Health Care in America: Essays in Social History*, ed. Susan Reverby and David Rosner (Philadelphia: Temple University Press, 1979), pp. 206–19, and Melosh,

"The Physician's Hand": Work Culture and Conflict in American Nursing (Philadelphia: Temple University Press, 1982).

3. Phrase from Elizabeth Marion Jamieson and Mary Sewall, *Trends in Nursing History: Their Relationship to World Events*, 2nd ed. (Philadelphia: W. B. Saunders, 1944; first published 1940), p. 295. Other major nursing histories include M. Adelaide Nutting and Lavinia L. Dock, *A History of Nursing*, 4 vols. (New York: G. P. Putnam, 1907–12); Mary M. Roberts, *American Nursing: History and Interpretation* (New York: Macmillan, 1954); Lucy Ridgeley Seymer, *A General History of Nursing*, 4th ed. (London: Faber and Faber, 1956; first published 1932); Lena Dixon Dietz, *History and Modern Nursing* (Philadelphia: F. A. Davis, 1963); Minnie Goodnow, *Nursing History*, 7th ed. (Philadelphia: W. B. Saunders, 1942; first published 1916).

4. "More General Staff Nurses," *American Journal of Nursing* (hereafter cited as *AJN*), 38 (April 1938): 30 (S); Beulah Amidon, *Better Nursing for America* (Public Affairs Pamphlets, No. 60; New York: Public Affairs Committee, 1941), pp. 13–14; Everett C. Hughes, Helen MacGill Hughes, and Irwin Deutscher, *Twenty Thousand Nurses Tell Their Story* (Philadelphia: Lippincott, 1958), p. 258.

5. Quotation from Temple Burling, Edith M. Lentz, and Robert N. Wilson, *The Give and Take in Hospitals* (New York: G. P. Putnam, 1956), p. 105.

6. For a humorous and perceptive analysis of the informal negotiations that mediate this new relationship, see Leonard I. Stein, "The Doctor–Nurse Game," *Archives of General Psychiatry* 16 (June 1967): 699–703. For examples of the recognition of nurses' roles in medical work culture, see Doctor X, *Intern* (New York: Harper & Row, 1965); Elizabeth Morgan, *The Making of a Woman Surgeon* (New York: G. P. Putnam, 1980); the 1955 film *Not as a Stranger*, based on the Morton Thompson novel of the same name, in which a senior doctor counsels his intern, "Make friends with the nurses. They run the hospital."

7. Interview with Astrid N., Oct. 23, 1976.

8. For an excellent review of the rapid diffusion of this reorganization and related medical technology, see Louise B. Russell, "The Diffusion of New Hospital Technologies in the United States," *International Journal of Health Services* 6:4 (1976): 557–580. For contemporary reports on these innovative units and on progressive patient care, see "Post-Anesthesia Unit at Presbyterian Hospital," *Trained Nurse and Hospital Review* (hereafter cited as *TNHR*), 121 (October 1948): 196; "Special Care Unit for Seriously Ill Patients," *Nursing World* (hereafter cited as *NW*) 130 (December 1956): 6; J. Murray Beardsley, M.D. and Florence Carvisiglia, R.N., "A Special Care Ward for Surgical Patients," *NW* 131 (March 1957): 11–13; Edward J. Thomas, "Progressive Patient Care," *NW* 134 (March 1960): 11–12, 32. Early reports often emphasized the use of this reorganization to alleviate the nursing shortage by making more effective use of nurses. As

Louise B. Russell reports, however, this expectation was not borne out, since special care units required such high nurse–patient ratios. For recent discussions of the close working relations of doctors and nurses in intensive care, see Jon Franklin and Alan Doelp, *Shocktrauma* (New York: St. Martin's Press, 1980) and B. D. Colen, *Born at Risk* (New York: St. Martin's Press, 1981).

9. For evidence of private duty nurses' resistance to home cases, see May Ayers Burgess, *Nurses, Patients, and Pocketbooks: Report of a Study of the Economics of Nursing* (New York: Committee on the Grading of Nursing Schools, 1928), p. 98; "The Registry Looks at the Private Duty Nurse," *AJN* 29 (December 1929): 1465; "Our Mutual Obligation to Nursing," *AJN* 38 (February 1938): 193; Mary Louise Habel and Doris Milton, *The Graduate Nurse in the Home* (Philadelphia: Lippincott, 1939), p. vii.

10. Quotation from Elizabeth Maury Dean, "One Hundred Who Were Private Duty Nurses," *AJN* 44 (June 1944): 560.

11. The Red Cross voluntary aides ultimately became a source of wartime recruitment for paid auxiliaries, as discussed in "Red Cross Aides May Be Employed by Hospitals," *AJN* 44 (May 1944): 502; and Ida M. MacDonald, R.N., "Nurse's Aides for the Army," *AJN* 44 (July 1944): 659–60. For a statistical report of the widespread use of paid auxiliaries during the war, see Louise M. Tattershall and Marion E. Attenderfer, "Paid Auxiliary Nursing Workers Employed in General Hospitals," *AJN* 44 (August 1944): 752–56.

12. For nurses' complaints about the pace and division of labor in hospitals, see, for example, J. M. G. (probably Janet M. Geister), "An Open Letter on Staff Nursing," *TNHR* 106 (April 1941): 362; "Staff Nursing as It Is?" letter in *AJN* 41 (December 1941): 1448; "Administratively Speaking—Our Readers Write Us," *AJN* 41 (October 1941): 1176; letter from R.N., Aberdeen, Wash., *R.N.* 1 (July 1938): 3–4.

13. "Tribute to an American War Nurse," *Army Nurse* 1 (July 1944): 5; Victor Robinson, *White Caps: The Story of Nursing* (Philadelphia: Lippincott, 1946), p. 358. In an intriguing memoir, army nurse Edith A. Aynes describes her battles with the war public-relations bureau. She wanted the nurse presented as a professional; the bureau explicitly sought to show the nurse as a woman and "morale booster." See *From Nightingale to Eagle* (Englewood Cliffs, N.J.: Prentice-Hall, 1973), p. 257. For a broader discussion of women's work in World War II, see Leila Rupp, *Mobilizing Women for War: German and American Propaganda, 1939–1945* (Princeton, N.J.: Princeton University Press, 1978) and Karen Anderson, *Wartime Women: Sex Roles, Family Relations, and the Status of Women During World War II* (Westport, Conn.: Greenwood Press, 1981).

14. For information on patterns of women's participation in the labor force, see Janet Hooks, *Women's Occupations Through Seven Decades* (Washington: Zenger Publishing Co., 1978) and Valerie Kincade Oppenheimer, *The Female Labor Force in the United States: Demographic and*

Economic Factors Governing Its Growth and Changing Composition (Berkeley: University of California Population Monograph Series No. 5, 1970).

15.   Richard R. Lanese, *Authoritarianism in Nurses: Hospital-Significant Attitudes and Nursing Performance* (Columbus, Ohio: Systems Research Group, Engineering Experiment Station, 1961), pp. 42–43.

16.   T. K. Brown, "A Drink of Water," *O. Henry Awards Prize Stories, 1958* (Garden City, N.Y.: Doubleday, 1958), pp. 179–201; quotation from p. 199.

17.   David Charlson, *Night Nurse* (New York: Venus Books, 1951), pp. 31, 65, 68, 72.

18.   One well-known short story that represents a private duty nurse as outside "normal" marriage and sexuality is Dorothy Parker's "Horsie," in *After Such Pleasures* (New York: Harper & Row, 1958; story written in the 1920s), pp. 3–34. For stories that identify socially marginal nurses with sexual excess, see John Erskine, *Unfinished Business* (Indianapolis: Bobbs-Merrill, 1931); Conrad Aiken, "Bring! Bring!" in *The Collected Stories of Conrad Aiken* (Cleveland: World Publishing Co., 1960; first published in 1925 volume of the same name, *Bring! Bring!*); and Aiken, "The Night Before Prohibition,". in *The Collected Stories*, first published in *Among the Lost People*, 1934. For sociological interview, see Hughes, et al., *Twenty Thousand Nurses*, 191–92.

19.   Jane Converse, *Nurse Forrester's Secret* (New York: Signet, 1965), pp. 11–12; Helen Ashton [Jordan], *Yeoman's Hospital* (New York: Viking, 1945), p. 227; Arthur Gordon, "Old Ironpuss," *Saturday Evening Post*, May 12, 1951, pp. 149–53.

20.   Hans O. Mauksch, "Becoming a Nurse: A Selective View," *Medicine and Society*, special issue of *The Annals of the American Academy of Political and Social Science* 346 (March 1963): 88–98.

21.   Diane Frazer, *First Year Nurse* (New York: Pocket Books, 1964), pp. 40–41; Marguerite Mooers Marshall, *Wilderness Nurse* (New York: Pocket Books, 1960; first published 1949), pp. 47, 46.

22.   Kathleen Harris, *Jane Arden, Surgery Nurse* (New York: Popular Library, 1958), p. 123; Kathryn Morgan, *Tired Feet: The Story of a Registered Nurse* (New York: Vantage, 1952), p. 113; Marshall, *Wilderness Nurse*, p. 37; Peggy Gaddis, *Big City Nurse* (New York: McFadden, 1956), p. 6.

23.   Marshall, *Wilderness Nurse*, p. 201.

24.   Katharine Densford and Millard S. Everett, *Ethics for Modern Nurses: Professional Adjustments I* (Philadelphia: W. B. Saunders, 1947), pp. 198–99; Mary Price Smith, R.N., "A Day in the Life of Miss June Reynolds, Senior Nursing Student and 1950 Campus Queen," *NW* 124 (July 1950): 320–21; Theresa G. Muller, "Let's Talk It Over," *NW* 133 (May 1959): 28–29.

25.   Lucile Petry, in introduction to Densford and Everett, *Ethics for Modern Nurses*, p. iii; Zillah K. McDonald, *A Cap for Corrine* (New York:

Julian Messner, 1952), pp. 6, 8; Helen Wells, *Cherry Ames, Flight Nurse* (New York: Grosset and Dunlap, 1945), p. 305. In oral memoirs nurses trained in the 1940s and 1950s remembered hearing that nurses make good wives and mothers; interviews with Astrid N., Oct. 23, 1976; Anna D., Oct. 25, 1976, and Lorraine S., Oct. 26, 1976. In *To Work and to Wed: Female Employment, Feminism, and the Great Depression* (Westport, Conn.: Greenwood Press, 1980), Lois Scharf suggests that the pressure of negative public opinion helped to push defenders of married working women into retreat: they were forced onto narrow grounds. I think these changes in the postwar prescriptive literature show a similar retreat on the part of those who advised nurses.

9

Nursing Historiography, 1960–1980: An Annotated Bibliography

Mary Ann Dzuback

The literature of nursing history is rich in primary and secondary materials. Inspired in large measure by Adelaide Nutting's and Lavinia Dock's four-volume *History of Nursing*, scholars have examined the premodern practice of nursing, the emergence of professional nursing in the nineteenth and twentieth centuries, and the lives of notable nurses.

Until relatively recently the Nutting–Dock paradigm has dominated the historiography, with contemporary professional concerns providing standards of relevance within the field. Since the middle-1960s, however, historians have begun to raise new and more searching questions, to focus on a variety of fresh issues, and to place the particulars of nursing history within broader social, economic, political, and cross-cultural contexts.

Changes in the historiography of nursing pose interesting, important, and difficult questions for a bibliographer. What is nursing history? How far does this special field overlap with other related fields of history? Which works in sociology, in economics, in organizational theory have sufficient relevance to nursing history to warrant their inclusion in a bibliography such as this one? While raised at the outset, these questions shall not be answered by the material cited or the comments offered here. Faced with a choice of establishing more or less arbitrary boundaries or following clearly recognizable lines of demarcation, it has seemed sensible to follow the second course. By focusing on works that explicitly and centrally deal with nurses and nursing, with the places in which nurses have studied and worked, and with the organizations, causes, and events that have been of direct importance to nurses and to the structures that have defined their work as nurses, one may at least hope to delineate the core of the field. Further, within such relatively clear perimeters, the central categories of the field are more readily apparent and may implicitly serve to suggest the questions, perspectives, and peripheral literatures that historians have and have not yet begun to probe.

This bibliography shall categorize, cite, and comment upon studies in the history of nursing that have been published between 1960 and 1980 and that deal with nursing in the United States. Therefore it does not include such important guides to the literature as Virginia Henderson's *Nursing Studies Index*, 4 vols. (Philadelphia: J. B. Lippincott), which covers the years 1900–1959; Anne L. Austin's *History of Nursing Source Book* (New York: G. P. Putnam, 1957); and Bonnie Bullough's *Nursing: A Historical Bibliography* (New York: Garland, 1981). In addition, it does not include such general and organizational histories published prior to 1960 as Richard Shryock's *The History of Nursing: An Interpretation of the Social and Medical Factors Involved* (Philadelphia: W. B. Saunders, 1959) and Portia B. Kernodle's *The Red Cross in Action, 1882–1948* (New York: Harper & Bros., 1949).

A number of rich life stories published before 1960 also have been excluded—for example, Mary Breckinridge's *Wide Neighborhoods: A Story of the Frontier Nursing Service* (New York: Harper & Bros., 1952); Linda Richards's *Reminiscences of Linda Richards, America's First Trained Nurse* (Boston: Whitcomb & Barrows, 1911); Esther A. Werminghaus's *Annie W. Goodrich: Her Journey to Yale* (New York: Macmillan, 1950); and Sarah Tarleton Colvin's *A Rebel in Thought* (New York: Island Press, 1944).

Post-1980 studies, even those that are of critical importance to the field, do not appear here. Therefore studies like Susan Reverby's "The Nursing Disorder: A Critical History of the Hospital-Nursing Relationship, 1860–1945" (Ph.D. dissertation, Boston University, 1982), Mary P. Donahue's "Isabel Maitland Stewart's Philosophy of Education" (Ph.D. dissertation, University of Iowa, 1981), and Barbara Melosh's *"The Physician's Hand": Work Culture and Conflict in American Nursing* (Philadelphia: Temple University Press, 1982) are not cited in the following bibliography.

Despite the increasing importance of comparative studies, this bibliography considers only studies of nursing in the United States. Therefore works on Florence Nightingale and British nursing are excluded— for example, W. J. Bishop's and Sue Goldie's *A Biobibliography of Florence Nightingale* (London: Dawson's of Pall Mall, 1962); E. Huxley's *Florence Nightingale* (New York: G. P. Putnam, 1975); Elaine Showalter's "Florence Nightingale's Feminist Complaint: Women, Religion, and *Suggestions for Thought*" (*Signs* 6, Spring 1981); Brian Abel-Smith's *A History of the Nursing Profession* (London: Heinemann, 1960); and Celia Davies's *Rewriting Nursing History* (London: Croom Helm, 1980). Huda Abu-Saad's *Nursing: A World View* (St. Louis: C. V. Mosby, 1979), although not included here, briefly and simply provides accounts of the history of nursing in countries all over the world.

This bibliography is *not* intended to be all-inclusive; however, it does include many of the major works of synthesis that have appeared during the twenty years from 1960 to 1980, as well as a number of more specialized monographic studies.

Following a description of several major archive centers and general guides, five categories of literature shall be presented. Inevitably some works fall into a number of categories, but all have been grouped according to their central focus or major concentration.

I. ARCHIVE CENTERS AND GUIDES

Unfortunately there is no comprehensive guide to all the nursing archives in the United States. However, reference librarians at the major archive centers are helpful in making available the collections for which they are responsible and in directing scholars to other repositories.

Archive centers vary in the materials they have collected. For example, the Nursing Archive at Boston University's Mugar Memorial Library holds various institutional and organizational papers, including those of a number of hospitals and journals, and the personal papers, letters, and memorabilia of many of nursing's leaders. By contrast the *American Journal of Nursing*'s Sophia F. Palmer Memorial Library holds a large collection of books, periodical volumes, and pamphlets.

Many institutions that offer nursing education, the Pennsylvania Hospital for example, hold institutional records as well as journals and books. Some, notably the Archives at Teachers College, Columbia University, which include the Adelaide Nutting Historical Nursing Collection along with an extensive assortment of published materials and records of the Teachers College Division of Nursing Education, offer materials unavailable elsewhere in the world. The Hampton Institute School of Nursing in Hampton, Virginia, houses the M. Elizabeth Carnegie Nursing Archives, a growing collection that includes such diverse holdings as District 10 of the Virginia Nurses Association materials, the official repository for Chi Eta Phi (a sorority of black nurses), and a collection of oral, institutional, and personal historical materials with a focus on black nurses. Medical libraries, such as the National Library of Medicine and the Johns Hopkins University's Welch Medical Library, also often contain primary materials that are invaluable for nursing research.

Philanthropic organizations that have funded the development of nursing are yet another source of archival material. For example, the Rockefeller Archive Center in Pocantico Hills, New York, holds a great deal of material. The records of the Rockefeller Foundation are there and they contain project files on grants to nursing and medical education, midwifery programs, and hospitals around the world, as well as correspondence, grant administration, program, and policy reports. In addition, the Archive Center contains manuscripts related to Rockefeller-funded public health programs and other projects in which nurses worked. The Archive Center's most recent publication related to the history of nursing is *A Survey of Manuscript Sources for the History of Nursing and Nursing Education in the Rockefeller Archive Center, 1981.*

Among the available guides to nursing literature are the *International Nursing Index*, 15 vols., edited by Lucille Notter (New York: American Journal of Nursing, 1966–80), and the *Cumulative Guide to Nursing and Allied Health Literature*, 25 vols., edited by Mildred Grandbois and Ferne Fanning (Glendale, Calif.: Seventh-Day Adventist Hospital Association, 1956–80).

II. GENERAL HISTORIES

General nursing histories tend to recount the chronological development of nursing, often beginning with primitive healing practices and concluding with the current state of nursing. Many of them have been written as texts and, given their wide temporal scope, inevitably provide a rather superficial overview of the history. Acknowledging that nursing did not develop in a vacuum, works of this kind often peruse the history of civilization along with the history of nursing. Despite their tendency to sacrifice depth for coverage and to emphasize nursing's accomplishments and progress, these general histories do offer a great deal of basic factual information and straightforward chronological syntheses. They make available the "notable" people, activities, events, and turning points that have been fundamental to reconstructions of the past, and many provide extremely useful guides to other sources.

Occasionally one finds general histories that place recurring issues in a new light, that raise new issues, or that cover an unplumbed area of nursing history. Thus Bullough and Bullough (1964) provide background on persistent problems for the profession: low status, subordination to organized medicine, establishing universal training paradigms, and overcoming the constraints of gender-associated prejudices; Strauss (1965) describes past strategies for fostering the professionalization of nursing; Bullough and Bullough (1971) trace the economic problems of nurses, and the dilemmas that have been associated with sex-role expectations, professional control, and militant activities since World War II; and Kalisch and Kalisch (1978), in their most recent work, include a detailed examination of the problems facing minorities in American nursing.

Most general works of synthesis present the chronological development of nursing with little or no analysis or critique. Hence they imply that any new development in nursing has fostered "progress"—a step forward for nurses, nursing, and American society. Celia Davies (1980) offers suggestions concerning ways in which a reexamination of approaches to nursing history might stimulate more critical inquiries.

Books

BULLOUGH, VERN L. and BULLOUGH, BONNIE. *The Care of the Sick: The Emergence of Modern Nursing.* New York: Prodist, 1978.
  Provides a thorough survey of nursing history and touches on such recent historical issues as professional specialization, hierarchical stratification, and collective bargaining.

BULLOUGH, VERN L. and BULLOUGH, BONNIE. *The Emergence of Modern Nursing.* 2nd ed. London: Macmillan Co., 1969.
  Follows a survey format and chronicles professionalization with a concentration on education, associations, and leaders, and includes references to male and black nurses.

DELOUGHERY, GRACE. *History and Trends of Professional Nursing.* 8th ed. St. Louis: C. V. Mosby Co., 1977.
  Textbook.

DIETZ, LENE DIXON. *History and Modern Nursing.* Philadelphia: F. A. Davis Co., 1963.
  Textbook.

DOLAN, JOSEPHINE. *History of Nursing.* 12th ed. Philadelphia: W. B. Saunders, 1968.

A standard text in substance and style that includes recent developments in nursing history.

————. *Nursing in Society: A Historical Perspective.* 14th ed. Philadelphia: W. B. Saunders, 1968.
Emphasizes the influence on nursing of medical science, changing social attitudes, and religion, and includes an extensive bibliography.

GRIFFIN, GERALD and GRIFFIN, H. JOANNE KING. *Jensen's History and Trends of Professional Nursing.* 5th ed. St. Louis: C. V. Mosby Co., 1965.
Chronicles in textbook style the development of nursing.

HENDERSON, VIRGINIA and NITE, GLADYS. *The Principles and Practice of Nursing.* 6th ed. New York: Macmillan, 1978.
The first chapter (pp. 4–109) contains a survey of the history within the context of the authors' concerns for nursing practice.

JAMIESON, ELIZABETH M., SEWALL, MARY F., and SUHRIE, ELEANOR B. *Trends in Nursing History: Their Social, International, and Ethical Relationships.* 6th ed. Philadelphia: W. B. Saunders, 1966.
A general presentation of the history that includes an unusually extensive bibliography.

JOHNSTON, DOROTHY F. *History and Trends of Practical Nursing.* St. Louis: C. V. Mosby Co., 1966.
Specifically deals with the development of practical nursing, and considers the effects of the Goldmark Report—a study of nurse training schools—on the professionalization of both practical and registered nursing.

KALISCH, PHILIP and KALISCH, BEATRICE. *The Advance of American Nursing.* Boston: Little, Brown and Company, 1978.
See p. 185.

SANNER, MARGARET. *Trends and Professional Adjustments in Nursing.* Philadelphia: W. B. Saunders, 1962.
Textbook.

STEWART, ISABEL M. and AUSTIN, ANNE L. *A History of Nursing.* 5th ed. New York: G. P. Putnam, 1962.
Recounts the history of nursing in the United States, details the development of nursing in Canada, and offers a general survey of the international development of nursing.

STRAUSS, ANSELM. "The Structure and Ideology of American Nursing." In *The Nursing Profession: Five Sociological Essays,* edited by Fred Davis, pp. 60–108. New York: John Wiley & Sons, 1965.
See p. 185.

TINKHAM, CATHERINE W. and VOORHIES, ELEANOR F. *Community Health Nursing: Evolution and Process.* New York: Appleton-Century-Crofts, 1972.
Reviews the history of public health nursing within the context of the

history of nursing and suggests some of the outcomes of political and economic actions as they have influenced public health nursing.

Periodicals

BULLOUGH, VERN and BULLOUGH, BONNIE. "Nursing and History." *Nursing Outlook* 12 (October 1964): 27–29.
 See p. 185.

———. "The Origins of Modern American Nursing: The Civil War Era." *Nursing Forum* 2:2 (1963):13–27.
 A cursory probe into the beginnings of professional nursing.

CHRISTY, TERESA E. "The Fateful Decade, 1890–1900." *American Journal of Nursing* 75 (July 1975): 1163–65.
 Concentrates on one ten-year period of nursing history and supplies a detailed list of nursing leaders.

DAVIES, CELIA. "Where Next for Nursing History?" *Nursing Times* 76 (May 22, 1980): 920–22.
 See p. 185.

FITZPATRICK, M. LOUISE. "Nurses in American History: Nursing and the Great Depression." *American Journal of Nursing* 75 (December 1975): 2188–90.
 Relates the changes wrought in the profession during the depression.

———. "Nursing." *Signs* 2 (Summer 1977): 818ff.
 Provides historical background on current problems in the profession and offers interesting contrasts with other articles in this issue, which was devoted to an examination of women's careers.

GABRIELSON, ROSAMOND C. "Two Centuries of Advancement: From Untrained Servant to Skilled Practitioner." *Journal of Advanced Nursing* 1 (July 1976): 265-72.
 Emphasizes the professional growth of American nursing since the Civil War.

HENDERSON, VIRGINIA. "Excellence in Nursing." *American Journal of Nursing* 69 (October 1969): 2133–37.
 Presents Henderson's definition of excellence within a historical context.

SHRYOCK, RICHARD. "Nursing Emerges as a Profession: The American Experience." *Clio Medica* 3 (May 1968): 131–47.
 Focuses on American nursing, American attitudes toward women, and the effects of those attitudes on professionalization and the development of nursing in relation to the development of the medical profession (also in Leavitt and Numbers, pp. 203–15; see p. 199).

III. NURSING EDUCATION

Histories that deal with nursing education tend to examine the organizational characteristics of institutions involved in nursing education as well as the impact of specific institutions on the development of nursing education throughout the United States. The broadening focus of educational history to include such nonschool agencies of education as the church, the family, and the media does not seem to have been taken into full account by historians of nursing.

Prior to the 1960s there were a number of training-school histories that set the pattern for later institutional studies—a pattern that, once again, exhibits a great concern for places, dates, major personalities, and "progress." During the 1970s, however, some studies of individual training schools began to consider the immediate and more enduring influences of school requirements and how those requirements were related to ideological positions within the profession. For example, Tomes (1978) not only provides an intensive examination of the internal administration, operation, and life of one hospital training school, she also analyzes the ideological framework manifest in the authority of the school's superintendent, the moral and social characters of its students, and the relationship between the school and its associated hospital. In that way she delineates the nature of the opportunities that attracted women, who were searching for a professional identity, into nursing. Mottus (1980) provides another in-depth historical analysis of nurse training, in this instance via an account of two hospital training schools and the far-reaching and powerful influences on nursing and medical care of their curricula, their graduates, and their policies. She reveals internal conflicts between the training schools and their hospital affiliations, and her unprecedented profiles of the schools' students include abundant statistical information on the women and men who participated in the training schools' programs.

Books

Brown, Janie M. "Master's Education in Nursing, 1945–1969." In *Historical Studies in Nursing*, edited by M. Louise Fitzpatrick, pp. 104–30. New York: Teachers College Press, 1978.

Explores nursing educators' efforts to establish, develop, and fund post-graduate degree programs for nurses.

CHRISTY, TERESA E. *Cornerstone for Nursing Education.* New York: Teachers College Press, 1969.
Details the development of graduate education for nurses at Teachers College and explores the influence of Teachers College graduates, personnel, and programs on the nursing profession and on women's status in public positions.

FADDIS, MARGENE O. *A School of Nursing Comes of Age: A History of the Francis Payne Bolton School of Nursing, Case Western Reserve University.* Cleveland, Ohio: The Alumnae Association of the Francis Payne Bolton School of Nursing, 1973.

GRAY, JAMES. *Education for Nursing: A History of the University of Minnesota School.* Minneapolis: University of Minnesota Press, 1960.
Relates the unique story of nursing educators and education at the University of Minnesota, an institution that encouraged and supported nursing education for women.

HEISTAD, WANDA. "The Development of Nurse-Midwifery Education in the United States." In *Historical Studies in Nursing,* edited by M. Louise Fitzpatrick, pp. 86–103. New York: Teachers College Press, 1978.
Condensed from her dissertation (see p. 191).

LEE, ELEANOR. *Neighbors, 1892–1967.* New York: Columbia University–Presbyterian Hospital School of Nursing Alumnae Association, 1967.

MacDONALD, GWENDOLINE. *Development of Standards and Accreditation in Collegiate Nursing Education.* New York: Teachers College Press, 1965.
Examines some of the factors affecting nursing education and the accreditation of nursing educational institutions.

MOTTUS, JANE E. *New York Nightingales: The Emergence of the Nursing Profession at Bellevue and New York Hospitals, 1850–1920.* Ann Arbor, Mich.: UMI Research Press, 1980.
See p. 188.

PERKINS, SYLVIA. *A Centennial Review: The Massachusetts General Hospital School of Nursing, 1873–1973.* Boston: School of Nursing, Nurses Alumnae Association, 1975.
Provides a detailed chronological history of the school—its development, external associations, internal reorganizations, ongoing operation, and numerous directors.

SLOAN, PATRICIA. "Commitment to Equality: A View of Early Black Nursing Schools." In *Historical Studies in Nursing,* edited by M. Louise Fitzpatrick, pp. 68–85. New York: Teachers College Press, 1968.
Abridgement of dissertation (see p. 193).

Periodicals

ABDELLAH, FAYE G. "Evolution of Nursing as a Profession." *International Nursing Review* 19:3 (1972): 219–38.
> Recounts the development of the nursing profession and the various professional studies that influenced educational emphases over time.

BAYLDON, MARGARET O., ed. "Diploma Schools: The First Century." *RN* 36 (February 1973): 33.
> Provides a short chronological history of various training schools and examines changes that resulted from the increasing demands of the American Nurses' Association for collegiate nursing programs.

BULLOUGH, BONNIE and BULLOUGH, VERN. "Collegiate Nursing in the United States—An Historical Review." *International Nursing Review* 10 (January/February 1963): 41–47.
> A brief survey of obstacles and incentives to nursing education as it grew within colleges and universities.

CHRISTY, TERESA E. "Clinical Practice as a Function of Nursing Education: An Historical Analysis." *Nursing Outlook* 28 (August 1980): 493–97.
> Presents the conflict within training schools between educating nursing students and servicing the needs of hospitals.

————. "Entry into Practice: A Recurring Issue in Nursing History." *American Journal of Nursing* 80 (March 1980): 485–88.
> Investigates the financial dependence of early training schools on their hospital affiliations and the exchange of service for sponsorship between the schools and the hospitals.

DOLAN, JOSEPHINE. "Three Schools—1873." *American Journal of Nursing* 75 (June 1975): 989–92.
> Explores the contrasts among three United States training schools that were originally based on the Nightingale Plan.

DREVES, KATHERINE D. "Nurses in American History: Vassar Training Camp for Nurses." *American Journal of Nursing* 75 (November 1975): 2000–2002.
> Details the organization of the camp and its daily operation.

GOWAN, M. O. "Influence of Graduate Nurses on the Formative Years of a University School of Nursing. A Memoir." *Nursing Research* 16 (Summer 1967): 261–66.
> A brief history of the Catholic University School of Nursing.

KALISCH, BEATRICE J. and KALISCH, PHILIP A. "Slaves, Servants, or Saints? (An Analysis of the System of Nurse Training in the United States, 1873–1948)." *Nursing Forum* 14:3 (1975): 222–63.
> Examines the Nightingale Plan in England, its importation to the United

States, and its subsequent transformations in response to social, political, and professional pressures.

RAWNSLEY, MARILYN M. "The Goldmark Report: Midpoint in Nursing History." *Nursing Outlook* 21 (June 1973): 380–83.

Provides a brief analysis of the Goldmark Report—a study of nurse training programs—and its influence in altering the pattern of nursing education.

SHARP, BENITA HALL. "The Beginnings of Nursing Education in the United States: An Analysis of the Times." *Journal of Nursing Education* 12 (April 1973): 26–32.

Sketches the social climate within which the first training schools were established in the United States.

TOMES, NANCY. "Little World of Our Own: The Pennsylvania Hospital Training School for Nurses, 1895–1907." *Journal of the History of Medicine and Allied Sciences* 33 (October 1978): 507–30.

See p. 188.

Dissertations

ALLEMANG, MARGARET MARY. "Nursing Education in the United States and Canada, 1873–1950: Leading Figures, Forces, Views on Education." Ph.D. dissertation, University of Washington, 1974.

Through the ideas of nursing leaders, Allemang explores the formation of nursing education in both countries in light of intellectual and social forces for change, and how those ideas constantly were reconceptualized.

BROWN, BILLYE JEAN. "The Historical Development of the University of Texas System School of Nursing, 1890–1973." Ed.D. dissertation, Baylor University, 1975.

CASWELL, ELEANOR. "Historical Study of Emotional Support and the Patterns of Teaching Roles of the General Duty Nurse, 1900–1970." Ed.D. dissertation, Boston University, 1971.

CHAPMAN, MURIEL ELIZABETH. "Nursing Education and the Movement for Higher Education for Women: A Study in Interrelationships, 1870–1900." Ed.D. dissertation, Columbia University, 1969.

Explores relationships between the expansion of higher education for women and the growth and proliferation of training schools for nurses.

HEISTAD, WANDA CAROLINE. "Midwife to Nurse-Midwife: A History. The Development of Nurse-Midwifery Education in the Continental United States to 1965." Ed.D. dissertation, Teachers College, Columbia University, 1977.

Describes the rise and decline of plans to establish nurse-midwife training programs and the effects of changing priorities in nursing education on the profession of midwifery.

HOFFMAN, M. MARIAN KASABIAN. "The Beginnings of Basic Baccalaureate Nursing Education: 1916–1929." Ph.D. dissertation, Ohio State University, 1968.
Examines three universities to explore the forces and groups that encouraged or hampered the establishment of baccalaureate programs in nursing.

HOLLAND, HOWARD OWEN. "Historical Survey of Attendant-Nurse Training in Michigan." Ph.D. dissertation, Michigan State University, 1974.

JOHNSON, HELEN R. "A History of Purdue University's Education Programs." Ed.D. dissertation, Indiana University, 1975.

KRAMPITZ, SYDNEY DIANE. "The Historical Development of Baccalaureate Nursing Education in the American University: 1899–1935." Ph.D. dissertation, University of Chicago, 1978.
An examination of seven undergraduate programs.

LABECKI, GERALDINE. "Baccalaureate Programs in Nursing in the Southern Region. 1925–1960." Ed.D. dissertation, George Peabody College for Teachers, 1967.

LAWRENCE, CORA JANE. "University Education for Nursing in Seattle, 1912–1950: An Inside Story of the University of Washington." Ph.D. dissertation, 1972.

NOALL, SANDRA HAWKES. "A History of Nursing Education in Utah." Ed.D. dissertation, University of Utah, 1969.
Describes the origins and growth of nursing education in Utah as one community's response to shifting emphases in professional nursing.

NOROIAN, ELIZABETH LLOYD. "The School of Nursing of the University of Pittsburgh: 1939–1973." Ph.D. dissertation, University of Pittsburgh, 1980.
Delineates the establishment, curriculum development, and ultimate state affiliation of the school within the context of local and national influences and needs.

PARIETTI, ELIZABETH SHELVIN. "The Development of Doctoral Education for Nurses: An Historical Survey." Ed.D. dissertation, Teachers College, Columbia University, 1979.

PAYLOR, MARY MARGARET. "A History of Nursing Education in Florida from 1893–1970." Ph.D. dissertation, Florida State University, 1975.

SHEAHAN, DOROTHY ALICE. "The Social Origins of American Nursing and Its Movement into the University: A Microscopic Approach." Ph.D. dissertation. New York University, 1979.
Examines the Connecticut Training School and Yale University School of

Nursing to focus on the social groups that provided nursing and nurse training with its early character and the professional groups that changed that character through educational reform.

SLOAN, PATRICIA ELLEN. "A History of the Establishment and Early Development of Selected Nurse Training Schools for Afro-Americans: 1886–1906." Ed.D. dissertation, Teachers College, Columbia University, 1978.

Traces the establishment and lifespans of four training schools for black nurses and provides an analysis of the conditions that demanded their establishment, of efforts to maintain their standards, and of the factors that contributed to the eventual demise of three of the schools.

SMOLA, BONNIE KETCHUM. "A Study of the Development of Diploma and Baccalaureate Degree Nursing Education Programs in Iowa from 1907–1978." Ph.D. dissertation, Iowa State University, 1980.

Explores the influences of women and economic pressures on health delivery systems as well as the relationship between traditional medicine and nursing, and includes descriptions of the political activities of nursing leaders and organizations as they affected the development of nursing education in Iowa.

STORY, DONNA KETCHUM. "A Study of Practical and Associate Degree Nursing Education in Iowa from 1918–1978." Ph.D. dissertation, Iowa State University, 1980.

IV. NURSING PRACTICE

Nursing practice has been shaped by beliefs, attitudes, and customs, by historical events, discoveries, and people, by changing social structures, social institutions, and patterns of social organization, and of course by politics (see next category). In a sense nursing practice cannot be conceived as a distinct category within the historiography. The foregoing notwithstanding, however, some works do focus far more explicitly than others on how health care practices have been defined and changed over time. It is works of this kind that are grouped here.

More often than not, wars, epidemics, and disasters are stressed in studies that are attentive to changes in nursing practice. Therefore the kind of "thick description" that is increasingly evident in labor history has not yet become fully apparent in nursing history. Historians of nursing, especially in exploring maternal health and health care, have begun to incorporate more ecological perspectives drawn from the history of medicine and the history of women.

Books

ANTLER, JOYCE and FOX, DANIEL M. "The Movement Toward a Safe Maternity: Physician Accountability in New York City, 1915–1940." In *Sickness and Health in America: Readings in the History of Medicine and Public Health*, edited by Judith Walzer Leavitt and Ronald L. Numbers, pp. 375–92. Madison: University of Wisconsin Press, 1978.
> Examines the relationships among maternal health, public health services, and rising standards of medical practice and thus provides a useful perspective on the history of midwifery.

EHRENREICH, BARBARA and ENGLISH, DIERDRE. *Witches, Midwives, and Nurses: A History of Women Healers*. Old Westbury, N.Y.: The Feminist Press, 1973.
> Although a concentration on the oppression of women tends to accent women's roles as victims, this exploration of the involvement of women in the healing process presents a useful account of midwifery.

KOBRIN, FRANCES. "The American Midwife Controversy: A Crisis of Professionalization." In *Sickness and Health in America: Readings in the History of Medicine and Public Health*, edited by Judith Walzer Leavitt and Ronald L. Numbers, pp. 217–25. Madison: University of Wisconsin Press, 1978.
> Analyzes the factors that led to the increasing dominance of the medical profession in the field of maternal health and childbirth and examines statistics on infant mortality as well as public response to growing professional specialization in the field.

LITOFF, JUDITH B. *American Midwives: 1860 to the Present*. Westport, Conn.: Greenwood Press, 1978.
> An unusually clear and interesting narrative of the development of midwifery in the United States.

MASSEY, MARY ELIZABETH. *Bonnet Brigades*. New York: Knopf, 1966.
> Investigates nursing as one of the increasingly varied activities outside the home that were opened to women as a result of the Civil War.

PARKS, ROBERT J. *Medical Training in World War II*. Washington, D.C.: Office of the Surgeon General, Department of the Army, 1974.
> An analysis of training programs in the Army Nurse Corps that includes copious facts and figures.

Periodicals

"The Army Nurse." *American Journal of Nursing* 66 (February 1966): 290–92.
> Briefly outlines the history of the Army Nurse Corps.

AUSTIN, ANNE L. "Wartime Volunteers—1861–1865." *American Journal of Nursing* 75 (May 1975): 816–18.
Portrays the roles women assumed in response to the Civil War and the recognition they received for their organizational and nursing work.

BOGDAN, JANET. "Care or Cure? Childbirth Practices in Nineteenth Century America." *Feminist Studies* 4 (June 1978): 92–99.
Favorably contrasts the humane, experiential approaches to childbirth of midwives with the more theoretical and less personal approaches of physicians.

BULLOUGH, BONNIE. "The Lasting Impact of World War II on Nursing." *American Journal of Nursing* 76 (January 1976): 118–20.
Analyzes gender and racial integration in the Army Nurse Corps, the growing importance of trained people in the health services, and the increasing pressure toward hierarchical organization in civilian hospital nursing services.

GRIFFITH, WILLIAM and NEWCOMB, RICHARD. "The Nurse in America: The Image of a Century." *RN* 33 (February 1970): 37–57.
Provides a survey of Red Cross nursing in America, nursing during peacetime, and nursing during war.

GUYOT, SISTER HARRIET. "The Nurse in Civil War Literature." *Nursing Outlook* 10 (May 1962): 311–14.
Describes the growing consciousness of the need for trained nurses that made the Civil War a source of opportunity for women interested in assuming more public responsibilities.

HUGHES, SISTER ANN ELIZABETH; BERTONNEAU, SISTER DOROTHEA; and ENNA, CARL DEMIAN. "Nurses at Carville." *American Journal of Nursing* 68 (December 1968): 2564–69.
Briefly outlines the history of the leprosy colony in Louisiana and the contributions of the Sisters of Charity who nursed the lepers there.

KALISCH, BEATRICE J. and KALISCH, PHILIP A. "Be a Cadet Nurse: The Girl with a Future." *Nursing Outlook* 21 (July 1973): 444–49.
Analyzes the effects of publicity on the American public's awareness of the needs of and opportunities in army nursing.

————. "The Cadet Nurse Corps—in World War II." *American Journal of Nursing* 76 (February 1976): 240–42.
Chronicles the establishment of the Cadet Nurse Corps.

————. "Heroines of 98." *Nursing Research* 24 (November–December 1975): 411–29.
Describes the activities of nurses during the Spanish-American War and explains how those activities inspired the establishment of the Army Nurse Corps.

KALISCH, PHILIP A. and KALISCH, BEATRICE J. "Nurses Under Fire: World

War II Experiences of Nurses on Bataan and Corregidor." *Nursing Research* 25 (November–December 1976): 409–29.

———. "Untrained but Undaunted: The Women Nurses of the Blue and the Gray." *Nursing Forum* 15 (1976): 4–33.
Describes renowned and obscure Civil War nurses.

———. "The Women's Draft." *Nursing Research* 22 (September–October 1973): 402–13.
Criticizes government and military bureaucratic decisions and actions in regard to the proposed women's draft during World War II.

LITOFF, JUDY B. "Forgotten Women: American Midwives at the Turn of the Twentieth Century." *The Historian* (February 1978): 235–51.
Provides a detailed account of the practice of midwifery during a time when physicians were attempting to gain control of obstetrics and public health officials were struggling to establish training for midwives.

SELAVAN, IDA C. "Nurses in American History: The Revolution." *American Journal of Nursing* 75 (April 1975): 592–94.
A description of nursing work during the American Revolution.

TIRPAK, HELEN. "The Frontier Nursing Service—Fifty Years in the Mountains." *Nursing Outlook* 23 (May 1975): 308–10.
Provides a brief history with accompanying photographs.

WOOD, ANN DOUGLAS. "The War Within a War: Women Nurses in the Union Army." *Civil War History* 18 (September 1972): 197–212.
Reflecting a historiographical concern for women's struggles for recognition in society, this article illustrates how women, in their confrontations with military and medical authorities, improved the health and welfare of soldiers and turned medical incompetence into a professional opportunity for themselves.

Dissertations

CALIANDRO, GLORIA GAYLE BROWN. "The Visiting Nurse Movement in the Borough of Manhattan, New York City, 1877–1917." Ed.D. dissertation, Teachers College, Columbia University, 1970.
Traces the development of the movement and its connections with various organizations, industry, and educational institutions.

MELOSH, BARBARA. "'Skilled Hands, Cool Heads, and Warm Hearts': Nurses and Nursing, 1920–1960." Ph.D. dissertation, Brown University, 1979.
Probes numerous histories—of medicine, society, women, and labor—to apply a historical and sociological critique to concepts of the development of the profession. Melosh effectively communicates a sense of nurses' experiences in private duty, public health, and hospital nursing.

REGAN, PATRICIA ANN. "An Historical Study of the Nurse's Role in School Health Programs from 1902–1973." Ed.D. dissertation, Boston University School of Education, 1974.

Examines the changing functions of school nurses in relation to various perspectives on disease, health education, and nursing education.

SNIHUROWYCZ, MARIA ZORESLAWA. "The Frontier Nursing Service of Kentucky and Its Antecedents in Public Health Nursing." Ph.D. dissertation, Yale University, 1968.

TIRPAK, HELEN. "The Frontier Nursing Service: An Adventure in the Delivery of Health Care." Ph.D. dissertation, University of Pittsburgh, 1972.

A history of the service that covers its development, administration, financial organization, and health care practices.

V. NURSING POLITICS AND FEMINISM: QUESTIONS OF POWER AND CONTROL

Historical studies having to do with nursing politics are distinguishable by their concern with questions of power and control. In works of this kind the growth of the nursing profession, as a profession, has been emphasized. As portrayed in most accounts, professional nursing organizations have played an important role in nursing politics via their attempts to initiate and maintain control of the professionalization process through the supervision of standards and accreditations in nursing education and the establishment and maintenance of graduate-nurse licensing procedures. Of course, other factors have also encouraged nurses' attempts to assume and maintain control of their work. For example, positive attitudes toward women and work and nurses' involvement in feminist activities have also been politically significant, and they too are studied in the kinds of works grouped together here. In addition there are studies that deal with developments within the medical profession, particularly when those have impinged directly upon the development of the nursing profession, or have influenced attitudes toward nurses within hospitals and other institutional settings.

Although most analyses of nursing politics portray change as progress deriving from a series of politically beneficial cause-and-effect relationships, some works are more critical in their analyses of organizational activity and institutional milieu. Thus Fitzpatrick (1975) defines the scope of the National Organization for Public Health Nursing and provides an analysis of the strengths and weaknesses that have affected its development and eventual decline; Cannings and Lazonick (1975) illuminate questions of control as implicit in professional developments, especially within the areas of education and legislation for licensing; Reverby (1979) probes hospital management, nurse training, and nursing services within hospitals to present the thesis that nurses have worked to reinforce hospital hierarchies in order to facilitate the smooth functioning of hospitals and to secure their own positions within those hierarchies; and Ashley (1977) explores the coincidence of hospital proliferation with the development of the nursing profession—the point being to examine nurses' subordination to and dependence on physicians' control of patient care and their paradoxical support for hospitals within and over which, according to Ashley, they have had little power or control.

Books

Ashley, Jo Ann. *Hospitals, Paternalism, and the Role of the Nurse.* New York: Teachers College Press, 1977.
   See above.

Baker, Elizabeth Faulkner. *Technology and Women's Work.* New York: Columbia University Press, 1964.
   Provides a short history of the nursing profession, including its connection with Nightingale's work, within the context of women's work in a technological society.

Bridges, Daisy Caroline. *A History of the International Council of Nurses, 1899–1964.* Philadelphia: J. B. Lippincott Co., 1967.
   Documents the formation, meetings, and agendas of the International Council of Nurses.

Brown, Esther Lucille. "Nursing and Patient Care." In *The Nursing Profession: Five Sociological Essays,* edited by Fred Davis, pp. 176–202. New York: Wiley & Sons, 1965.
   Examines tensions present in nurses' perceptions of patient care and the actual activities involved in nursing practice as these relate to the teaching of middle-class values that was inherent to early nurse training programs, and raises questions concerned with nurses' loss of autonomy as patient care has become more institutionalized within hospitals.

Brownlee, W. Elliot and Brownlee, Mary M. *Women in the American Economy: A Documentary History, 1675–1929.* New Haven: Yale University Press, 1976.
   Explores the ways, including nursing, in which women have contributed to the American economy, and further examines political and social factors contributing to women's particular occupational choices.

DRISCOLL, VERONICA M. *Legitimizing the Profession of Nursing: The Distinct Mission of the New York State Nurses Association.* New York: New York State Nurses Association, 1976.
> Describes the association's efforts to realize and maintain legislation licensing the practice of nursing and to retain a voice in and control of the licensing process. Explores how the association helped to define and legitimate the profession.

DUFFY, JOHN. *A History of Public Health in New York City, 1625–1866.* New York: Russell Sage Foundation, 1968.
> Provides a comprehensive and detailed study of the growth of public health consciousness in New York and examines immigration, sanitation, and the development of medicine and hospitals as they have contributed to public health care. In addition Duffy describes the conditions contributing to the later development of nursing.

FITZPATRICK, M. LOUISE. *The National Organization for Public Health Nursing, 1912–1952: Development of a Practice Field.* New York: National League for Nursing, 1975.
> See p. 197.

FLANAGAN, LYNDIA, COMP. *One Strong Voice: The Story of the American Nurses' Association.* Kansas City, Mo.: The American Nurses' Association, 1976.
> The principal historical study of the American Nurses' Association and its major accomplishments.

KESSLER-HARRIS, ALICE. "Women, Work, and the Social Order." In *Liberating Women's History*, edited by Berenice A. Carroll, pp. 330–43. Urbana: University of Illinois Press, 1976.
> Ties economics into the rationale behind attitudes toward women in the work force during the eighteenth and nineteenth centuries and describes women's efforts to develop training programs, professional attitudes, and careers in the professions and "semi-professions," such as nursing.

LEAVITT, JUDITH WALZER and NUMBERS, RONALD L., eds. *Sickness and Health in America: Readings in the History of Medicine and Public Health.* Madison: University of Wisconsin Press, 1978.

REVERBY, SUSAN. "Health Is Women's Work." In *America's Working Women: A Documentary History, 1600 to the Present*, compiled and edited by Rosalyn Baxandall, Linda Gordon, and Susan Reverby, pp. 346–50. New York: Vintage Books, 1976.
> Presents a short chronological history of nursing in light of economic pressures on the profession from growing paramedical specializations and practical nursing.

——. "The Search for the Hospital Yardstick: Nursing and the Rationalization of Hospital Work." In *Health Care in America*, edited by Susan

Reverby and David Rosner, pp. 206–19. Philadelphia: Temple University Press, 1979.

See p. 198.

—— and ROSNER, DAVID, eds. *Health Care in America*. Philadelphia: Temple University Press, 1979.

ROSEN, GEORGE. *Preventive Medicine in the United States, 1900–1975*. New York: Science History Publications, 1975.

Analyzes preventive medicine within the context of public health and social legislation, much of which was influenced by nurses.

ROSENBERG, CHARLES. *The Cholera Years*. Chicago: University of Chicago Press, 1972.

Deals with the effects of cholera epidemics in nineteenth-century America, examines societal attitudes toward disease and public health, and mentions the Sisters of Charity as the only organized nursing group available to respond to the epidemics.

——. "The Therapeutic Revolution: Medicine, Meaning, and Social Change in Nineteenth-Century America." In *The Therapeutic Revolution*, edited by Morris J. Vogel and Charles E. Rosenberg, pp. 3–25. Philadelphia: University of Pennsylvania Press, 1979.

Examines social and medical attitudes toward illness and health during the period that nursing was emerging as a profession.

ROTHMAN, SHEILA. *Woman's Proper Place: A History of Changing Ideals and Practices, 1870 to the Present*. New York: Basic Books, 1978.

Depicts the complex interrelationships among women's professions (including nursing), women's rights, and societal pressures and mores, and examines these interrelationships in terms of the adjustments and compromises women and society have made to women's increasing activities in such areas as public health nursing and nurse training.

SHRYOCK, RICHARD H. *Medicine and Society in America, 1660–1860*. New York: New York University Press, 1960.

Studies the influences of English medicine on American medicine and explores cultural attitudes, scientific developments, and early attempts to upgrade custodial nursing, as they have related to medicine, hospitals, and public health.

SMUTS, ROBERT W. *Women and Work in America*. New York: Columbia University Press, 1960.

Chronicles the development of nursing within the larger context of women's work and compares nursing with other work available to women.

VOGEL, MORRIS J. *The Invention of the Modern Hospital*. Chicago: University of Chicago Press, 1980.

Studies the development of hospitals in Boston and correlates the changing functions and services of the hospital with the advances and priorities of medicine and physicians and with the increasing urbanization of American society, again providing background on the period during which nursing was emerging as a profession.

————. "Machine Politics and Medical Care: The City Hospital at the Turn of the Century." In *The Therapeutic Revolution*, edited by Morris J. Vogel and Charles E. Rosenberg, pp. 159–75. Philadelphia: University of Pennsylvania Press, 1979.

Examines the political machinations behind conflicting perceptions of the primary purpose of the hospital—physicians' views of the hospital as a place for research and study and the public's view of the hospital as a place for the care of the indigent, the eventual outcome of which was a greater community acceptance of hospitals that contributed to an increased demand for nursing within hospitals.

————. "Patrons, Practitioners, and Patients: The Voluntary Hospital in Mid-Victorian Boston." In *Sickness and Health in America: Readings in the History of Medicine and Public Health*, edited by Judith Walzer Leavitt and Ronald L. Numbers, pp. 173–84. Madison: University of Wisconsin Press, 1978.

Provides a glimpse of nineteenth-century Boston hospitals, from the perspective of the patients who patronized them, during the period prior to and including the emergence of professional nurse training.

————. "The Transformation of the American Hospital: 1850–1920." In *Health Care in America*, edited by Susan Reverby and David Rosner, pp. 105–10. Philadelphia: Temple University Press, 1979.

Explores the turn-of-the-century shift from home to hospital care of the ill and offers background on the social attitudes that have affected nurses' positions within hospital health care.

WERTHEIMER, BARBARA M. *We Were There: The Story of Working Women in America*. New York: Pantheon Books, 1977.

Provides an overview of women's contributions to all facets of economic life throughout American history and presents nursing as an example of a field in which women have utilized their organizational abilities to establish a profession and to respond to social need.

Periodicals

"AJN 1900–1975." *American Journal of Nursing* 75 (October 1975): 1609–14. Photographic essay.

ARNOLD, VIRGINIA. "The Past: Way to the Future." *International Nursing Review* 21 (May–August 1974): 68–76.

Presents a short history of the International Council of Nurses.

ASHLEY, JO ANN. "Nursing and Early Feminism." *American Journal of Nursing* 75 (September 1975): 1465–67.
  Portrays the failure of nurses to control their own education and practice in relation to their support of male-dominated hospital institutions.

BRAND, KAREN L. and GLASS, LAURIE K. "Perils and Parallels of Women and Nursing." *Nursing Forum* 14:2 (1975): 160–74.
  Places the nursing profession within the framework of women's professions and interests.

BULLOUGH, BONNIE. "The New Militancy in Nursing." *Nursing Forum* 10:3 (1971): 273–88.
  Focuses on nurses' militancy by tracing nurses' economic problems and examining sex-role expectations and how these have related to nurses' control of their working conditions.

CANNINGS, KATHLEEN and LAZONICK, WILLIAM. "The Development of the Nursing Labor Force in the United States: A Basic Analysis." *International Journal of Health Services* 5:2 (1975): 185–216.
  See p. 197.

CARNEGIE, MARY ELIZABETH. "The Path We Tread." *International Nursing Review* 9 (September–October 1962): 25–33.
  Presents the employment and training problems of black nurses in American history.

——— and OSBORN, ESTELLE. "Integration in Professional Nursing." *International Nursing Review* 9 (August 1962): 47–50.
  Briefly surveys racial integration in professional nursing organizations.

CHRISTY, TERESA. "Equal Rights for Women: Voices from the Past." *American Journal of Nursing* 71 (February 1971): 288–93.
  Describes the various political factions and professional groups within nursing that supported or opposed voting rights for women.

———. "The First Fifty Years." *American Journal of Nursing* 71 (September 1971): 1778–84.
  Briefly details the internal functioning of the American Nurses' Association as it responded to external events over which it had little control.

ELMORE, JOYCE ANN. "Black Nurses: Their Service and Their Struggle." *American Journal of Nursing* 76 (March 1976): 435–37.
  Sketches black nurses' activities in terms of forming their own professional organizations and their eventual acceptance into mainstream nursing.

"From ANA's Album." *American Journal of Nursing* 71 (September 1971): 1774–77.
  Collection of photographs from 1896 through 1970.

INGLES, THELMA. "The Physicians' View of the Evolving Nursing Profession." *Nursing Forum* 15:2 (1975): 123.

Deals with physicians' responses to nursing from 1873 to 1913.

"ICN Presidents: Leaders Who Have Forged the Future." *International Nursing Review* 21 (May–August 1974): 77–110.

In addition to this photographic essay of the leaders of the International Council of Nurses, this issue presents a number of articles commemorating the history of the ICN.

KALISCH, PHILIP A. "How Army Nurses Became Officers." *Nursing Research* 25 (May–June 1976): 164–77.

Describes the lobbying efforts of nurses and political leaders to achieve passage of a bill requiring the ranking of nurses in the army.

LEMONS, J. STANLEY. "The Sheppard-Towner Act: Progressivism in the 1920s." *Journal of American History* 55 (March 1969): 776–86.

Examines the needs for and the effects of the Sheppard-Towner Act.

———. "Social Feminism in the 1920s: Progressive Women and Industrial Legislation." *Labor History* 14 (Winter 1973): 83–91.

Provides a perspective on the women involved in promoting child labor laws, one of the activities in which politically concerned nurses were interested.

MOORE, MARY LOU. "Bright Spot in the 18th Century." *American Journal of Nursing* 69 (August 1969): 1705–9.

Describes public health as the major concern in the design of an early American Moravian community and the political respect accorded male and female nurses for their contributions to community health.

MORANTZ, REGINA. "Making Women Modern: Middle Class Women and Health Reform in 19th Century America." *Journal of Social History* 10 (June 1977): 490–507.

Explores women's extra-familial activities that encouraged the Popular Health Movement and educated the public. Provides a perspective on the concerns of women from the middle class, from which many of nursings' early leaders emerged.

REVERBY, SUSAN. "Hospital Organizing in the 1950s: An Interview with Lillian Roberts." *Signs* 1 (Summer 1976): 1053–63.

Presents the militant activities of hospital personnel other than administrators, doctors, and nurses, and mentions the support the strikers received from doctors and nurses.

ROBERTS, JOAN T. and THETIS, M. G. "The Women's Movement and Nursing." *Nursing Forum* 12:3 (1973): 303–22.

Examines women healers, the structure of doctor-nurse relationships, and nurses' attitudes toward the women's movement.

ROSENBERG, CHARLES. "And Heal the Sick: The Hospital and the Patient in 19th Century America." *Journal of Social History* 10 (June 1977): 428–47.

Examines public attitudes toward hospitals and describes evolving modes of patient care during the period in which nursing was emerging as a profession.

————. "Social Class and Medical Care in Nineteenth-Century America: The Rise and Fall of the Dispensary." *Journal of the History of Medicine and Allied Sciences* 29 (January 1974): 32–54.
Studies medicine's shifting priorities in relation to disease and illness in the care of the indigent and to the increasing use of hospitals rather than dispensaries for that care. Also describes the functional roles visiting nurses assumed in association with the dispensaries.

ROSENCRANTZ, BARBARA. "Cart Before the Horse: Theory, Practice, and the Professional Image in American Public Health, 1870–1920." *Journal of the History of Medicine and Allied Sciences* 29 (January 1974): 55–73.
Explores the roles of physicians and public health boards and their alliances with public works departments in early disease prevention. Investigates the implications for doctor-nurse relationships and of changing medical attitudes toward disease and increasing reliance on hospitals.

SCHUTT, BARABARA G. "The Recent Past." *American Journal of Nursing* 71 (September 1971): 1785–91.
Examines structural changes in the American Nurses' Association and the ways that nurses have become more vocal about their working conditions.

SHANNON, MARY LUCILLE. "Our First Four Licensure Laws." *American Journal of Nursing* 75 (August 1975): 1327–29.
Illustrates the early work of professional associations as they endeavored to enact state licensure laws and thereby retain control of standards of professional nursing practice.

SMITH-ROSENBERG, CARROLL. "Politics and Culture in Women's History." *Feminist Studies* 6 (Spring 1980): 55–64.
Uses examples such as the Henry Street Settlement—a group of nurses who lived and worked in an immigrant neighborhood—to argue that the study of women's history requires an examination of the cultural and social networks that women formed to initiate and empower their work in various fields, including nursing and politics.

WEILER, P. G. "Health–Manpower Dialectic–Physician, Nurse, Physician Assistant." *American Journal of Public Health* 65 (August 1975): 858–63.
A historical approach to the development of "roles" within the health professions.

ZIMMERMAN, ANNE. "ANA: Its Record on Social Issues." *American Journal of Nursing* 76 (April 1976): 588–90.
Provides an overview of various American Nurses' Association legislative concerns.

Dissertations

BYTHEWAY, RUTH EVON. "History of the Development of the Nursing Service of the Veteran's Administration under the Direction of Mrs. Mary A. Hickey, 1919–1942." Ed.D. dissertation, Teachers College, Columbia University, 1972.
 A study of the growth, development, and influence of the organization on nursing education and public health nursing.

DENTON, DAVID REHMI. "The Union Movement in American Hospitals, 1847–1976." Ph.D. dissertation, Boston University, 1976.
 Likens health care unions to the initial organization of the American Medical Association and the American Nurses' Association, and examines the histories of those organizations.

DICKENS, MARION RACHEL. "The Influence of the Position of Women on the Development of Nursing as a Profession in America." Ph.D. dissertation, University of New Mexico, 1977.

MAZERO, JEAN LOUISE. "Professionalizing of Nursing in America: A Century of Struggle." Ph.D. dissertation, University of Pittsburgh, 1972.
 Traces professional nursing's conceptual framework, as nursing has changed from its nineteenth-century origins as a "caring" profession to its twentieth-century classification as a "sub-profession," in relation to efforts to professionalize, the emergence of nursing education, and the commitment of the nursing profession to professional medicine and the public.

McMENEMY, AGNES CATHERINE. "The History of Collective Bargaining in Professional Nursing in Michigan." Ed.D. dissertation, Wayne State University, 1979.

PIEMONTE, ROBERT V. "A History of the National League of Nursing Education, 1912–1932: Great Awakening in Nursing Education." Ed.D. dissertation, Teachers College, Columbia University, 1976.
 Explores the development of that organization as it affected nursing education and, ultimately, nursing practice in the United States.

SCHISSEL, CARLA MAE. "The State Nurses' Association in a Georgia Context, 1907–1946." Ph.D. dissertation, Emory University, 1979.
 Focuses on one state nurses' organization as a microcosmic study of the development of professional nursing.

SWORT, ARLOWAYNE. "The ANA: The Formative Years, 1875–1922." Ed.D. dissertation, Teachers College, Columbia University, 1974.
 Examines the socioeconomic forces that contributed to the forming of a national association of nurses and the concerns within the organization

that influenced its increasing involvement in legislation to control professional and educational standards.

VI. LIVES

The number of available life histories of nurses, biographies, autobiographies, and memoirs, is enormous. Accounts of nurses' lives, in addition to presenting biographical data, provide substantial information about nurse education, nurse organizations and work settings, and general social conditions and conflicts. Occasionally they proceed well beyond the facts of a particular life to present an especially cogent analysis of a larger issue or problem.

For example, Schuyler (1975), in describing the activities of two nursing leaders, Florence Nightingale and Louisa Lee Schuyler, illuminates the ideological differences between two approaches to the professionalization of nurses. Henle (1978), in critically assessing Clara Barton's activities with the Red Cross, makes apparent Barton's hardly unique wish for a life of danger and excitement. Lagemann (1979), in analyzing the education of Lillian Wald, shows the way in which the constraints inherent in traditional nursing roles led Wald to settlement work and visiting nursing as vehicles through which to enact her interests and ideals. And James (1979), in studying Isabel Hampton, explicates the special significance of the Johns Hopkins Nurse Training School.

Books

AUSTIN, ANNE L. *The Woolsey Sisters of New York: 1860–1900*. Philadelphia: American Philosophical Society, 1971.
> Describes familial influences on the Woolseys, their nursing activities during the Civil War, their extended commitments to nurse training, hospital improvements, and social reform, and the importance of the support they derived from a network of social and medical relationships.

AYNES, E. *From Nightingale to Eagle: An Army Nurse's History*. Englewood Cliffs, N.J.: Prentice-Hall, 1973.
> Memoir of Aynes's training, service in the Army Nurse Corps, postgraduate study, and World War II duty.

CUNNINGHAM, JOHN T. *Clara Maas—A Nurse—A Hospital—A Story*. Cedar Grove, New Jersey: Rae, 1976.

GOOSTRAY, STELLA. *Memoirs of Half a Century in Nursing*. Boston: Nursing Archive, Boston University Mugar Memorial Library, 1969.

Recounts her training, teaching, administrative, and writing experiences and chronicles her involvements with other nursing leaders in pursuit of professionalization.

GREGG, ELINOR D. *The Indians and the Nurse*. Norman: University of Oklahoma Press, 1965.
An account of Gregg's work with Native Americans that illustrates the difficult conditions of rural district nursing and illuminates the ways that federal bureaucracies have deliberately controlled and limited public health services, particularly for minorities.

JAMES, EDWARD T., et al., eds. *Notable American Women, 1607–1950*, 3 vols. Cambridge, Mass.: Harvard University Press, 1971.
Presents concise accounts of the lives and accomplishments of many nursing leaders.

JAMES, JANET WILSON. "Isabel Hampton and the Professionalization of Nursing in the 1890s." In *The Therapeutic Revolution*, edited by Morris J. Vogel and Charles E. Rosenberg, pp. 201–44. Philadelphia: University of Pennsylvania Press, 1979.
See p. 206.

LAGEMANN, ELLEN CONDLIFFE. "Lillian D. Wald." In *A Generation of Women: Education in the Lives of Progressive Reformers*, pp. 59–86. Cambridge, Mass.: Harvard University Press, 1979.
See p. 206.

MARKS, GEOFFREY and BEATTY, WILLIAM K. *Women in White*. New York: Charles Scribner's Sons, 1972.
A collection of brief biographies.

MARSHALL, HELEN E. *Mary Adelaide Nutting, Pioneer of Modern Nursing*. Baltimore: Johns Hopkins University Press, 1972.
A chronological account of Nutting's life and accomplishments that reveals the importance of the supportive networks formed by nursing leaders and the degree to which Nutting's ambition to establish high educational standards for nurses was a widely shared ideal.

SAFIER, GWENDOLYN. *Contemporary American Leaders in Nursing: An Oral History*. New York: McGraw-Hill, 1977.
The histories and experiences of various nurses chosen by their colleagues to tell their stories.

SICHERMAN, BARBARA, et al., eds. *Notable American Women: The Modern Period*. Cambridge, Mass.: Harvard University Press, 1981.

STAUPERS, MABEL KEATON. *No Time for Prejudice: A Story of the Integration of Negroes in the United States*. New York: Macmillan, 1961.
Narrates the story of Staupers's life as a prominent leader of black nurses, particularly during World War II, within the context of the struggle of black nurses to develop training schools and an organization, the Na-

tional Association of Colored Graduate Nurses, to deal with employment discrimination against black nurses.

YOST, EDNA. *American Women of Nursing.* 3rd ed. Philadelphia: J. B. Lippincott Co., 1965.
Provides short, elementary biographies of twentieth-century nursing leaders.

Periodicals

ACHIWA, GORO. "Linda Richards in Japan." *American Journal of Nursing* 68 (August 1968): 1716–19.
Enumerates Richards's accomplishments in Japan and the outgrowth of her work there: the establishment of the Japanese Red Cross and of numerous training schools.

ALGER, GEORGE W. "Lillian D. Wald: An Artist in the Joy of Living." *American Journal of Nursing* 60 (March 1960): 354–57.
Recollection of Wald's work.

BROWN, HELEN E. "A Tribute to Mary Breckinridge." *Nursing Outlook* 10 (May 1962): 54–55.

CARBARY, LORRAINE. "Linda Richards: America's First Trained Nurse." *Journal of Practical Nursing* 23 (October 1973): 22–24.

CHRISTY, TERESA. "Portrait of a Leader: M. Adelaide Nutting." *Nursing Outlook* 17 (January 1969): 20–24.
Provides a brief account of Nutting's accomplishments and interests.

———. "Portrait of a Leader: Annie Warburton Goodrich." *Nursing Outlook* 18 (August 1970): 46.
Enumerates Goodrich's accomplishments in nursing, including her superintendency of the Army School of Nurses and the Yale School of Nursing.

———. "Portrait of a Leader: Isabel Hampton Robb." *Nursing Outlook* 17 (March 1969): 26.
Chronicles Robb's life, work, and publications.

———. "Portrait of a Leader: Isabel M. Stewart." *Nursing Outlook* 17 (October 1969): 44–48.
Presents Stewart's training, administrative work, and curriculum work in nursing at Teachers College.

———. "Portrait of a Leader: Lavinia Lloyd Dock." *Nursing Outlook* 17 (June 1969): 72–75.
Narrates Dock's early background, nurse training, political activities, and publications.

———. "Portrait of a Leader: Lillian D. Wald." *Nursing Outlook* 18 (March 1970): 50–54.

Retells the story of Wald's work at Henry Street, her work with visiting nurses, and her initiation of a system of public school nurses.

———. "Portrait of a Leader: Sophia F. Palmer." *Nursing Outlook* 23 (December 1975): 746–51.
Provides a short biographical account of Palmer's training and her work, particularly her initiation of the *American Journal of Nursing*.

CURTISS, JOHN. "Russian Nightingale." *American Journal of Nursing* 68 (May 1968): 1029–31.
Presents a glimpse of Russian nurses' experiences in the Crimean War through a short biography of one nurse—Ekaterina M. Bakunina.

DOCK, LAVINIA. "Lavinia L. Dock: Self-Portrait." *Nursing Outlook* 75 (January 1977): 23–26.
A previously unpublished recollection of Dock's nursing career and her political activities.

GEISTER, JANET. "This I Believe About My Life." *Nursing Outlook* 12 (March 1964): 58–61.
A memoir of Geister's work in public health and with the American Nurses' Association.

GOOSTRAY, STELLA. "Sophie Nelson: Public Health Statesman." *American Journal of Nursing* 60 (September 1960): 1268–69.

HENLE, ELLEN L. "Clara Barton—Soldier or Pacifist?" *Civil War History* 24 (June 1978): 152–60.
See p. 206.

KYLE, R. A. and SHAMPO, M. A. "Clara Louise Maas." *Journal of the American Medical Association* 244 (July 1980): 75.

MONTEIRO, LOIS A. "Lavinia L. Dock (1947) on Nurses and the Cold War." *Nursing Forum* 17:1 (1978): 46–54.
An annotated collection of Dock's letters to President Harry Truman that illustrates the international and political scope of her concerns for nursing.

OBLENSKY, FLORENCE. "Anita Newcombe McGee, M.D. (4 Nov. 1864–5 Oct. 1940)." *Military Medicine* 133 (May 1968): 397–400.
Recounts McGee's success as the founder of the Army Nurse Corps.

SELAVAN, IDA. "Bobba Hannah, Midwife." *American Journal of Nursing* 73 (April 1973): 681–83.
Traces the historical background of eastern European midwifery and describes the social and cultural spheres of midwifery in immigrant neighborhoods in American cities, through the life story of one midwife.

STEWART, ISABEL. "Recalls the Early Years." *American Journal of Nursing* 60 (October 1960): 1426–30.
A narrative of Stewart's training and work and of those of other nursing leaders.

Dissertations

DANIELS, DORIS. "Lillian D. Wald: The Progressive Woman and Feminism." Ph.D. dissertation, City University of New York, 1977.
   Analyzes Wald's progressive affiliations and feminist activities in relation to her accomplishments in nursing.

NOEL, NANCY LOUISE. "Isabel Hampton Robb: Architect of American Nursing." Ed.D. dissertation, Teachers College, Columbia University, 1979.
   Studies Robb's life and influence in the process of professionalization of nursing.

RESNICK, ALLAN EDWARD. "Lillian D. Wald: The Years at Henry Street." Ph.D. dissertation, University of Wisconsin, 1973.
   Examines Wald's life at Henry Street.

SCHUYLER, CONSTANCE BRADFORD. "Molders of Modern Nursing: Florence Nightingale and Louisa Lee Schuyler." Ed.D. dissertation, Teachers College, Columbia University, 1975.
   See p. 206.

About the Contributors

SUSAN ARMENY is a doctoral candidate in the history department of the University of Missouri-Columbia. She is writing a dissertation on the campaign to professionalize American nursing between 1893 and 1920.

JANE PACHT BRICKMAN has taught women's history and intellectual history at the United States Merchant Marine Academy, Hofstra University, Pace University, and Queens College of the City University of New York. Her Ph.D. dissertation was entitled "Mother Love, Mother Death. Maternal and Infant Care in Urban America: 1880–1930."

KAREN BUHLER-WILKERSON is a faculty member of the School of Nursing at the University of Pennsylvania. She is completing a Ph.D. dissertation in the Department of City Planning at the University of Pennsylvania on the history of public health nursing.

CELIA DAVIES is a senior research fellow in the Department of Sociology at the University of Warwick, Coventry, U.K. Her Ph.D. dissertation was a comparative study of nurse professionalization in Britain and the United States. She is editor of *Rewriting Nursing History*.

MARY ANN DZUBACK is a doctoral candidate in the Department of Philosophy and the Social Sciences at Teachers College, Columbia University.

ELLEN CONDLIFFE LAGEMANN is an associate professor of history and education at Teachers College, Columbia University, where she is also a research associate in the Institute of Philosophy and Politics of Education. She is the author of *A Generation of Women: Education in the Lives of Progressive Reformers* and of *Private Power for the Public Good: A History of the Carnegie Foundation for the Advancement of Teaching*.

BARBARA MELOSH is an assistant professor of history and women's studies at the University of Wisconsin–Madison. She has held research fellowships at the Smithsonian Institution in Washington, D.C. and is the author of *"The Physician's Hand": Work Culture and Conflict in American Nursing*.

SUSAN REVERBY is an assistant professor of women's studies at Wellesley College. Her Ph.D. dissertation was entitled "The Nursing Disorder: A Critical

211

History of the Hospital-Nursing Relationship, 1860–1945." She is a co-editor of *America's Working Women: A Documentary History* and of *Health Care in America: Essays in Social History.*

NANCY TOMES is an assistant professor of history at the State University of New York at Stony Brook and holds a postdoctoral fellowship in the Rutgers-Princeton Program in Mental Health Research, funded by the National Institute of Mental Health. She is the author of *A Generous Confidence: Thomas Story Kirkbride and the Art of Asylum Keeping 1840–1883.*

Index